Pediatric
Imaging

Pediatric Imaging

CECILIE GODDERIDGE, BS, RT(R)

Consultant and Lecturer in Pediatric Imaging
Formerly, Director, Education and Recruitment
Department of Radiology
Children's Hospital
Boston, Massachusetts

W.B. SAUNDERS COMPANY
A Division of Harcourt Brace & Company
Philadelphia London Toronto Montreal Sydney Tokyo

W.B. SAUNDERS COMPANY
A Division of Harcourt Brace & Company

The Curtis Center
Independence Square West
Philadelphia, Pennsylvania 19106

Library of Congress Cataloging-in-Publication Data

Godderidge, Cecilie.
    Pediatric imaging / Cecilie Godderidge. — 1st ed.
        p.   cm.
    ISBN 0-7216-4534-8
    1. Pediatric diagnostic imaging.   I. Title.
    [DNLM: 1. Diagnostic Imaging—in infancy & childhood.   WN 240 1995]
RJ51.D5G63   1995
618.92′00754—dc20
DNLM/DLC   94-12234

PEDIATRIC IMAGING   ISBN 0-7216-4534-8

Printed in United States of America

Last digit is the print number: 9   8   7   6   5   4   3   2   1

To John A. Kirkpatrick, Jr., MD, and John K. McCarey, Jr., whose compassion for children and dedication to pediatric radiology inspired us all.

To my family, who would have been proud.

Acknowledgments

First of all I would like to thank the radiographers at Children's Hospital, Boston, for their support and for humoring my requests that they look out for the perfect film of a particular injury or condition in a patient of just the right age and size. It is their imaging that illustrates this book.

I would like to thank all the radiologists who read chapters, often more than once, lent films, reviewed diagrams, and offered advice and encouragement as my spirits and pen flagged. To the following, for the extra time and special help they gave to this endeavor, goes my sincere appreciation: Drs. Carlo Buonomo, Taylor Chung, Robert Cleveland, John Emans, Thorne Griscom, Diego Jaramillo, Robert Lebowitz, Harriet Paltiel, Rita Teele, and S. Ted Treves.

I would like to thank my contributors for their willingness to share their expertise: MaryAnn Chin, Royal T. Davis, Linda Poznauskis, Linda Sorensen, and Keith J. Strauss.

Special thanks are due Robert Davis, whose skill and patience produced great photographs, and to Timothy, Sahara, Nicholas S., Kristen, Nicholas, Danielle, Marissa, and Tylor, the children of our staff, who endured being our models.

I would also like to thank James Koepfler for explaining the mysteries of moiré and ISIS topography; Miriam Geller, our librarian, for coming to the rescue in completing references; and Jim and Larry, our darkroom technicians, for their help in copying films. Finally, a big thank you to Liz Davis, who spent many hours deciphering, typing, and editing this manuscript. I couldn't have done it without her.

The problem with acknowledgments is the concern that someone will be inadvertently left out. My gratitude and thanks, therefore, go to all my colleagues. This book is about them, our patients, and the work we do in the department of radiology at Children's Hospital.

Preface

I have worked in pediatric radiography for over 30 years. As a staff radiographer I loved working with children, and being British-trained, I have had the opportunity to work with children on both sides of the Atlantic. Although eventually I became an administrative technologist and at various times have been an educator, it was my good fortune to be able to continue my career in a children's hospital.

I have given many lectures on pediatric radiography, and this book is a response to the questions and concerns encountered throughout the years. It is not a cookbook of pediatric radiographic positioning. In most instances, positioning children is not much different from positioning adults, although fewer images and different projections may be needed, depending on the condition and the age of the child.

I hope this book will have a wide appeal, but it has been written for radiographers who work primarily with adults and whose contact with children is limited. Children tend to be viewed as smaller versions of adults but in fact they are dynamic, constantly changing individuals, with their own specialized diseases and emotional needs. Radiographers who work with adults frequently ask, "How do you keep a child still?" My philosophy is, the more you know about a subject, the more interesting it is, and in the case of pediatric imaging, the more fun it is and therefore the better the result. If you understand the basic concepts of working with children, holding and immobilizing is frequently unnecessary.

Included are chapters on radiography, nuclear medicine imaging, ultrasound, CT, and MRI and discussions of how, in some instances, these techniques complement one another. Because children are considered to be at greater risk from ionizing radiation than adults are, there are chapters on radiation protection and radiation dose. My hope is that this book will not only be a reference on pediatric imaging for radiographers but also provide a better understanding of the pediatric patient.

CECILIE GODDERIDGE

Contributors

MaryAnn Chin, MBA, RT(R)
Section Chief of CT Scanner, Children's Hospital, Boston, Massachusetts
Preparation for Computed Tomography and Magnetic Resonance Imaging

Royal T. Davis, CNMT, ARRT
Educational Coordinator, Nuclear Medicine Technology Program, Massachusetts College of Pharmacy and Allied Health Sciences; Technical Director, Division of Nuclear Medicine, Children's Hospital, Boston, Massachusetts
Nuclear Medicine Imaging

Linda Poznauskis, BS, RT(R)
Technical Director, Department of Radiology, Children's Hospital, Boston, Massachusetts
Immobilization

Linda Sorensen, RDMS
Ultrasound Supervisor, Children's Hospital, Boston, Massachusetts
Pediatric Ultrasound

Keith J. Strauss, MSc, DABR, DABMP
Associate in Radiology, Harvard Medical School; Director, Radiology, Physics and Engineering, Children's Hospital, Boston, Massachusetts
Typical Radiation Exposures and Doses During Common Pediatric Examinations

Contents

Chapter 5

The Urinary System   59

Chapter 6

The Appendicular Skeleton   75

Chapter 7

The Spine   95

Chapter 8
The Pelvis and Hips 117

Chapter 9
The Skull. 129

Chapter 10
Immobilization. 145
Linda Poznauskis

Chapter 11
Preparation for Computed Tomography and Magnetic Resonance Imaging 159
MaryAnn Chin

Chapter 12

Nuclear Medicine Imaging 169

Royal T. Davis

Chapter 13

Pediatric Ultrasound 187

Linda Sorensen
Cecilie Godderidge

Chapter 14

Radiation Protection in Children......................... 199

Chapter 1

The Psychosocial Aspects of Working with Children

HISTORICAL BACKGROUND OF PEDIATRIC MEDICINE AND RADIOLOGY

The health of infants and children and their value to society varies depending on the culture and economic climate into which they are born.[1] In earlier times, children were considered the property of their parents, their employers, or the state. They were often subjected to indescribable cruelties in factories, in mines, and sometimes in their own homes. If they were orphaned or abandoned, their fate was the street or an almshouse.

As people's lifestyle improved, they could afford to become compassionate. The more institutions prospered, the more society's ills became apparent and demanded improvement.[1]

In the 18th century, the concept of child health care hardly existed.[2] Illness was often thought to be the work of evil spirits, and treatment was designed to purge both body and soul. When children were sick, they were treated the same as adults. Physicians treated patients of all ages with emetics, purges, sweating, and blistering.[2] If young patients survived the remedy, they usually survived the disease.

Sanitation was primitive; then as now, flies and mosquitoes were a nuisance, but no one realized they carried disease. Frequent epidemics of smallpox, diphtheria, scarlet fever, yellow fever, and measles frequently resulted in the death of several children in one family.[2]

In 1769, the first pediatric hospital (called the Dispensary for Sick Children) was established in London. It was for children who were orphaned or abandoned; it closed 12 years later for lack of financial support. In the United States, the first pediatric institution was the Children's Hospital of Philadelphia, established in 1855. Chicago Children's Hospital followed in 1865 and Boston's Children's Hospital in 1869.[1]

Children's Hospital in Boston was founded at a time of great social and economic need. Immigrants flooding into the country were poor and uneducated, and their living conditions were unsanitary and overcrowded. Chronic infections, particularly tuberculosis, were rampant, and children died at an alarming rate.

Pediatric medicine is a comparatively new specialty. The first permanent professor of pediatrics was Thomas Morgan Rotch at the Harvard Medical School. Established in 1893 as a professor of diseases in infants and children, he became professor of pediatrics in 1903. In 1910 he published *The Roentgen Method of Pediatrics*, the first textbook on Pediatric Radiology.[3]

Pediatric radiology and radiography developed slowly because of the inadequacies of the equipment. Many of the radiographs in Rotch's book are of the upper and lower limbs and the hips. The roentgen method was considered helpful in diagnosing congenital dislocation of the hips.[3] The radiographs are better than might be expected.

The radiographic plates of the chest and abdomen in Rotch's book are a little blurry because of the long exposure time. Ariel George, the first radiologist at Children's Hospital, radiographed an infant's abdomen at 7 seconds exposure time rather than 15 seconds, which resulted in marked improvement in detail.[3] This reduction in exposure time also meant that fewer patients had to be etherized (etherization was common in those early years).

Improvement in equipment was slow. Generators and exposure times were inadequate for "uncooperative" patients, and while radiology departments were established exclusively for children in many hospitals during the 1920's and 1930's, it was not until after World War II that pediatric radiology became established as a specialty.[4] It was 1945 before a second book on pediatric radiology was published, written by John Caffey of Babies Hospital in New York.[4]

With today's three-phase equipment, computerized technology, and fast film/

screen combinations, there is no diagnostic radiographic examination that cannot be performed on infants or children. Obtaining a good diagnostic radiograph depends more on technique and approaching the child rather than immobilization and long exposure times, the earlier concerns.

WORKING WITH CHILDREN IN THE HOSPITAL SETTING

Unfortunately, many radiographers more used to working with adults may approach children with a mixture of fear and apprehension. These emotions are easily communicated to a child whose feelings may be much the same when entering a radiology department. This situation can lead to tears and frustration, often resulting in an incomplete examination. Questions I am asked most often when lecturing on pediatric radiography are "How do you keep a child still?" and "How do you immobilize these (seemingly) difficult and uncooperative patients?" There is no formula, but patience and preparation can work wonders in making a child's visit to a radiology department a more pleasant experience for both the patient and staff.

Readers who are parents will understand the basic philosophy of the remainder of this chapter, though some of you may have difficulty disassociating yourselves from the thought that "this could be my child." If you find radiographing a sick child emotionally disturbing, you should, if possible, ask someone else to do it for you.

Because understanding the pediatric population depends on the age of the child, it is helpful to divide patients into the following age groups: neonates, infants, toddlers, preschool children, school-age children, and adolescents. It is important to remember, however, that children do not develop at the same rate, and there is no clear-cut division between the groups. Also, children regress emotionally when they are ill and undergoing stressful tests in unfamiliar surroundings. Cooperation from a child may depend on his or her previous experiences as well as on the severity of the illness.

"If a child is hurt or ill or has some condition which needs investigation or surgical intervention, the drama surrounding the physical needs often masks all others. It is easy for frantic parents, as well as busy hospital staff, to forget that Johnny with appendicitis is still Johnny. The fact that he has a bellyache requiring expert attention does not stop him from being the child he has always been, requiring all the kinds of attention he has always needed."[5]

This quote from *Your Growing Child*, by Leach, emphasizes that children have special needs and are not, as stated in the cliché, just little adults.

One further important point is that the staff must try and understand the emotions the parent or guardian is experiencing. The radiographer and the child need the support of parents to ensure a successful examination. Banning parents from entering a procedure room is nonproductive and creates stress for everyone concerned. As Leach states in her book, very young children are often more upset at being separated from parents and handled by strangers than they are by the procedures themselves.[5] Parents should be included in the preparation of their child for a procedure, and, when possible, they should be given a clearly defined role.

NEONATES

Human babies are helpless compared with other mammals. Their needs for warmth, food, and love are basic. Depending on the examination, wrapping a baby with its arms across its chest, sometimes called swaddling, imparts a feeling of warmth and security.

Babies become fretful and cry if they are cold, and it is important to realize that neonates (birth to 4 weeks), in particular, become hypothermic very quickly. If a baby needs to be uncovered for more than a few minutes during fluoroscopy, for example, a commercial warmer can be used. To avoid burns, be sure to follow closely the directions posted on the device. At Children's Hospital, warmers run on infrared lamps and are positioned at no less than 28 inches (71 cm) from the mattress. A 28-inch spacer is attached to the lamp to check the distance.

Thin, radiolucent sheeting (cotton or disposable) should always be placed between a baby and the table or cassette. Be sure there are no creases, as these will show up as artifacts on the films of these patients and will interfere with the diagnostic quality of the examination.

Babies cry when hungry, and both baby and parent will be exhausted if kept waiting after fasting. Keep this in mind when scheduling a procedure requiring an empty stomach, and make every effort to schedule the youngest patients at the beginning of a fluoroscopic session. A pacifier may be helpful for a time, but if its use is prolonged, the stomach may become full of air, and a bellyache only adds to the baby's misery.

If a baby is hungry because the mother has been unable to feed it, find a quiet place for her to do so before proceeding with a routine examination. The baby will then become drowsy, more content, and much more cooperative.

Rocking chairs are helpful when young patients must be sedated for longer, more specialized examinations, such as computed tomography or magnetic resonance imaging. Nursing divisions place them beside isolettes or cribs to assist in comforting or feeding babies; these chairs are an inexpensive addition to a radiology department. A warm, secure, dry, and preferably not hungry neonate or young baby will be a much more compliant patient.

INFANTS

As infants (birth to 12 months) develop, so does their awareness of people and surroundings. Mother becomes the recognized, beloved figure, and the baby, who was once easily picked up and cuddled by adoring friends and relatives, starts to protest at being handled by strangers. It is normal for an infant to cry when taken from its mother, especially in an unfamiliar radiography procedure room with strange objects and sounds.

Separation anxiety, fear of the dark, and fear of being left alone are usual before the end of the first year. It is reassuring to patients in this age group to let a mother stay with her young infant. Most hospitals now make arrangements for at least one parent to stay overnight. Studies have shown that prolonged psychological stress follows separation due to hospitalization. Thus there is no reason, except for pregnancy or a state law, to keep a mother out of the room during a routine radiographic procedure. I have also seen mothers become hysterical waiting outside a closed door listening to their screaming children.

TODDLERS

Toddlers (12 months to 3 years) are the least likely to be cooperative, and you should not expect them to be. This is the time when "No" is their most frequent response to any request. They are too young to understand the radiographic procedure, and the equipment is strange and frightening. Young children, having had vaccinations early in life, find people dressed in white synonymous with needle sticks. Thus we cannot expect them to keep still, especially because toddlers are rarely still when awake.

Children in this age group also need a great deal of reassurance. Speak calmly, quietly, and firmly. Allow them to keep a special toy with them. Sometimes a parent may threaten to leave the child if he or she misbehaves. Unfortunately, the only person this helps is the parent, who can then get out of earshot. Threats never work, and if the child needs to return for follow-up films, it will be difficult to get him or her to enter a radiology department again. When a toddler arrives, have the room, the technique, and the cassettes ready, and move quickly.

PRESCHOOL CHILDREN

The preschool years (3 to 6 years) are a wonderful stage. Children in this age group learn to walk and talk, demonstrating by degrees some measure of independence. They want to do things by themselves. It is a wonderful time, when they have make-believe games and imaginary friends. But this imaginary world can also be frightening to young children, particularly at night or when it is dark.

Children in this age group have a limited sense of time. A 3-year-old will ask "Are we there yet?" within only 5 minutes of embarking on a 4-hour trip. From a radiographic perspective, this is a large problem for a child who has to fast. These children should be scheduled as early in the day as possible. It is difficult for a mother to watch her child all the time and prevent him or her from sneaking a drink of juice or water. She will equally be surprised when you tell her that her child's stomach is not empty. If you have to schedule a procedure for the afternoon, let the child have a light breakfast at 6 a.m.

Preschoolers also take things literally. Hearing phrases such as "put to sleep" or "having a shot" may have serious connotations. Very young children will have heard about a pet that was "put to sleep" never to wake up, or that a shot means killing or dying. Be careful with your explanations, and keep them short and simple.

As children develop, so does their understanding. They like to have control over their surroundings, so ask for their help and give them a job to do. Show them the equipment and let them touch it. They are very trusting, and if a procedure is going to hurt, be honest and tell them in a nonnegative way. Emphasize the positive by saying, for example, "You can hold my hand as tight as you like," or "We are working as fast as we can," or, if a shot is needed, "It is like a little mosquito bite." Above all, do not lie. You will lose their trust, and they may not believe you again. This all takes time, but 5 minutes of preparation can mean a shorter, uneventful examination and no repeats.

"Bribery" as well as coaching is permitted. At Children's Hospital we give children stickers for doing a great job (whether or not they do so). And children love Band-Aids —the smallest hurt, not always seen by the naked eye, merits a Band-Aid, which they show off like a badge of honor.

SCHOOL-AGE CHILDREN

This group (6 to 12 years) accumulates a great wealth of knowledge and understanding of the world around them. Unless they are socially deprived, they develop good interactive skills and are helpful and friendly. If they have a congenital or developmental condition and have been coming to the hospital for a number of years, they might know more about their illness than you do.

Six-year-olds have a tendency to peer over their shoulders at you once you have positioned them, so strategically placed pictures help them maintain the correct position. With a little practice, 6- or 7-year-olds will usually hold their breath.

It is important to assess the individual needs of a child. Some children grow faster than others, so a 4-year-old may look more like a 7-year-old but developmentally is not yet able to cooperate. On the other hand, an older child may regress because of his or her illness. Never say "Don't be a baby." An older child may be enduring a chronic illness or pain that prevents him or her from attending school or playing with friends. A child with a debilitating illness often feels alone and left out, particularly because friends at this age are not always very understanding and can be thoughtlessly cruel.

In the preteen years, the human body starts to change and develop. Children in this age group are very modest. Respect this modesty; keep them covered, and give them the same privacy you would give adults. Young boys may fear castration when undergoing intimate procedures. Lying exposed on a table being prepared for a voiding cystourethrogram is discomforting for both males and females.

The *Journal of the Association for the Care of Children's Health* has published many studies related to the psychological responses of children to health care experiences and hospitalization. One study on computed tomography[6] showed that the most frequent complaints concerned needle sticks and being placed in an uncomfortable body position. Emotions included feeling funny, scared, or nervous; being alone; not being able to move; and feeling like a prisoner. One patient reported, "Sometimes I thought the circles may have sharp edges as it was moving and it might cut me."[6] This emphasizes how important it is to validate a child's understanding of a procedure.

Children ages 9 to 11 have a better understanding of the computed tomography procedure and can articulate what information should be given to them beforehand. Preparation should always take into account the cognitive level of a child, but minimally the child should be told or shown what a machine looks like, whether it will hurt, whether he or she will receive a shot, and if he or she has to keep still.

For most children, the hospital (including the Radiology Department) is a totally unfamiliar environment. All children, regardless of age or admission status, indicate that they need information of an emotional/supportive nature.[7]

In the computed tomography study there was a strong emphasis on having a parent present; children reported that "It feels better with someone there," "My father held my hand and calmed me down," or "It is hard to be still; a parent can help."[6]

ADOLESCENTS

Adolescence (13 years and over), the transition from childhood to adulthood, is marked by biological, social, and psychological development. It is important to look good and to be well. Teenagers tend to wear the same clothes, and any variation from the social norm makes them feel insecure. The increase in teenage suicides attests to the lowered self-esteem of many teenagers.

Adolescents tend to have chronic illnesses such as cystic fibrosis and asthma, to incur traumatic injuries, or to develop serious diseases that require prolonged hospitalizations. These diseases or illnesses may prevent them from keeping up with their studies, playing sports, dancing, attending the high school prom, or participating in other important social events. Because widely swinging emotions are typical in this age group, a strong reaction to a debilitating illness is to be expected.

An adolescent may be unfriendly to the point of insolence or may regress to more childish behavior. It is important to understand that adolescents' reaction to illness will be different than that of adults. A third of the patient population in a pediatric facility tends to be teenagers with special health problems, needs, and anxieties.

Most children's hospitals have special programs and facilities for this age group. A general hospital will place teenagers with adult patients, an incompatible situation at best. Patients in adult wards tend to be very sick and elderly, which younger patients find depressing. Adolescent patients are more likely to want to watch television, have more telephone calls, and socially interact with young friends.

Teenagers may worry about radiation and its effect on their sexuality or on childbearing. Some may act "cool" and try to distance themselves from what is being done to them. Others may fuss and cry. While this behavior may be difficult to understand, in the long run these patients may cope better with their illness than those who are withdrawn. Whatever their strategy, remember that this 150-pound patient may look like an adult but is not one, so do not expect adult concerns and behavior.

Pregnancy may be an issue. Teenage girls frequently do not admit to being pregnant until they reach the radiology department. Some states require a radiographer to ask females over the age of 11 years if they might be pregnant before proceeding with a radiographic procedure. If there is hesitancy rather than denial, the follow-up question should be, "Are you sexually active? If so, are you taking precautions?" If the patient is sexually active and takes no precautions, contact the referring physician before proceeding with the examination.

In an emergency, it may be necessary to proceed (on the advice of a physician) with a limited examination. The patient's mother, who may be in the waiting room, is probably unaware of the situation, making it imperative that the girl's physician become involved to take care of the social implications of a teenage pregnancy.

Some teenagers are emancipated minors, living away from home and financially independent, or are married or unmarried and caring for a child. Even though under the age of consent, depending on state law, many have control of their own health care. Those who have children are responsible for raising them and for making decisions regarding their children's health and treatment. If a parent or guardian of any age is judged to be incompetent, then a court must decide what is to be done in the best interest of the child.

Children have rights. (See "Bill of Rights for Children and Teens," by the Association for the Care of Children's Health, at the end of this chapter.) Be familiar with the laws of the state in which you work. It is usual and customary to require written and informed consent from a parent or guardian before proceeding with an interventional procedure. Do not assume that your patient, although a teenager, has no say in his or her health care. Teenagers of any age should participate in decisions being made about their treatment.

Drugs and sexually transmitted diseases, including AIDS, are now a part of life for many adolescents. Teenagers may not have to worry about paying the rent or keeping a job, but they are concerned with physical appearances, playing a particular sport, or belonging to a group. A debilitating illness sets them apart. While some may be fortunate enough to have supportive friends, others may be left alone if their peers cannot cope with someone who no longer seems to be one of them.

OVERALL PERSPECTIVE FOR THE RADIOGRAPHER

When a child is ill, the entire family is affected. Parents are acutely aware that they have a responsibility to act in the best interest of their child. In many instances, the decisions that are made may affect the quality of life for their child not only in the present, but also in his or her adulthood.

A mother called me one day because her 2-year-old child, who had a severe respiratory infection, had had radiographs of the chest and upper airway. That morning the mother had listened to a radio program describing the dangers of x irradiation, particularly radiation to the thyroid. In the 1940's and 1950's this type of radiation was used therapeutically to reduce the size of the thymus gland. For an hour I tried to reassure her that what the program had described was a therapeutic dose of radiation and that the risk of thyroid cancer from a diagnostic chest x-ray was almost negligible. Her guilt and anxiety were compounded by the fact that the examination was negative. She felt that she should never have let her child be x-rayed. This anecdote demonstrates that the knowledge most people acquire about radiation from the radio, newspapers, and magazines is often misleading. The mother's guilt, although we might think it irrational, was real, and she thought that her actions might result in her child's getting thyroid cancer as an adult.

Advocates for patient relations at Children's Hospital continually emphasize that lack of communication is responsible for most of the misunderstanding, anxiety, and anger of many parents visiting a hospital. Parents are intimidated by hospital jargon, everyone is in a hurry, perceptions may be wrong, and they are confused about whom they can talk to. Tell parents what you are going to do, and encourage them to ask questions if they do not understand. The chest radiograph may be routine for the radiographer, but for the parent it may be one examination in a series of tests to rule out a serious illness.

Be sensitive to people of different cultural and religious backgrounds. They may view illness and treatment methods differently. As a workforce we are becoming more culturally diverse. Patients and their families, many of whom may not speak or understand English, need to know that hospital staff is acting in the best interest of their child.

The Joint Commission for the Accreditation of Healthcare Organizations, in its accreditation manual for 1993, in the section *Diagnostic Radiology Services*, states that staff must demonstrate the knowledge and skills necessary to provide care appropriate to the age of the patients they serve.[8]

The rationale for patient-age-specific job requirements relates to the unique physical and psychological needs of patients in specific age groups. For example, patients in the pediatric age groups often have not yet developed the ability to fully understand the treatment being administered. In addition, they may not possess the communication skills to describe clearly their reactions or responses to treatment. Such patients frequently express themselves nonverbally. Consequently, staff who assess, treat, or care for these patients should be able to understand their unique needs. For instance, they should be able to interpret nonverbal communication.[8]

Caring for adolescent or geriatric patients presents different challenges. For example, involving adolescents in the treatment process requires an understanding that the authoritarian approach probably will not be successful.[8]

This chapter can only be a brief overview of how to relate to children in a radiology department. There are many books and articles on children and hospitalization. The Association for the Care of Children's Health conducted a research project in the 1980's to answer the following question: "When a child life program is designed and implemented on the basis of theory and research, will it make a positive difference for children and parents?"[9] The association's manual, *Psychosocial Care of Children in Hospitals*,[9] published in 1990, was based on this study. Although it focuses primarily on the hospitalized child, the book is a good resource for any health care provider.

Each child and age group has particular anxieties and concerns. It is up to the radiographer to provide an understanding, supportive, and compassionate environment.

Bill of Rights for Children and Teens

In this hospital you and your family have the right to:

- Respect and personal dignity
- Care that supports you and your family
- Information you can understand
- Quality health care
- Emotional support
- Care that respects your need to grow, play, and learn
- Make choices and decisions

Respect and Personal Dignity

- You are important. We want to get to know you.
- We will tell you who we are, and we will call you by your name. We will take time to listen to you.
- We won't talk about you in your room or outside your door unless you know what is happening.
- We will honor your privacy.

Care that Supports You and Your Family

- You and your family are important. We will work together to make you as safe and comfortable as possible.
- All families are different. We want to learn about what's important to you and your family.
- There will be a place for a member of your family to spend the night in the hospital with you or near you.

Information You Can Understand

- We will explain things to you. We will speak in ways you can understand. You can ask about what is happening to you and why.
- Someone who speaks your language will help explain things to you.
- Someone from your family can be with you when people in the hospital are explaining things to you.

Quality Health Care

- You will be taken care of by doctors, nurses, and other people who know about children and teenagers.
- You have the right to know all of the people who take care of you in the hospital. You and your family can meet with them to plan what is best for you.
- We will work together with you and your family to make your stay in the hospital as short and as comfortable as possible.

Emotional Support

- When you are in the hospital, you might feel scared, mad, lonely, or sad. You can let people know how you feel. It is okay to cry or complain.
- You can have your family with you as much as possible. When this is not possible, the other people caring for you will explain why.

Continued on the following page

<hr>

Bill of Rights for Children and Teens *(Continued)*

- We can help you meet children and families who have had experiences like yours.
- You can wear your own clothing most of the time and keep your special things with you.
- You can talk or play with people who know how to help when you have questions or problems.
- You can ask to be moved to another room if you are uncomfortable or unhappy.

Care That Respects Your Need to Grow, Play, and Learn

- We will consider all your interests and needs, not just those related to your illness or disability.
- You have the right to rest, to play, and to learn. We will make sure that you have places and times for the things children your age need to grow and learn.

Make Choices and Decisions

- Your ideas and feelings about how you want to be cared for are important.
- You can tell us how we can help you feel more comfortable.
- You can tell us how you want to take part in your care.
- You can make choices whenever possible. Sometimes you can help decide when and where you get your treatments.

Adapted with permission of the Association for the Care of Children's Health, 7910 Woodmont Avenue, Suite 300, Bethesda, Maryland, 20814.

REFERENCES

1. Snedeker, L., One Hundred Years at Children's, The Children's Hospital, Boston, 1969
2. Cone, T.E. Jr., History of American Pediatrics, Little, Brown & Company, Boston, 1979
3. Rotch, T.M., The Roentgen Method of Pediatrics, J.B. Lippincott Company, Philadelphia, 1910
4. Caffey, J., The first sixty years of pediatric roentgenology in the United States 1896–1956, American Journal of Roentgenology, 76(3):437–454, 1956
5. Leach, P., Your Growing Child, 2nd ed., Alfred A. Knopf, New York, 1986
6. Cerreto, M., Hellier, A., Ptak, H., CATS inside my brain: Children's understanding of the cerebral computed tomography scan procedure, Children's Health Care Journal of the Association for the Care of Children's Health, 14(4):211–217, 1986
7. Gillis, A.J., Hospital Preparation: The Children's Story, Children's Health Care Journal of the Association for the Care of Children's Health, 1:19–27, 1990
8. Joint Commission for the Accreditation of Healthcare Organizations, Accreditation Manual For Hospitals, JCAHO, Oakbrook Terrace, IL, 1993
9. The Association for the Care of Children's Health, Psychosocial Care of Children in Hospitals, ACCH, Bethesda, MD, 1990

Chapter 2

The Chest

DEVELOPMENT OF THE RESPIRATORY SYSTEM

The respiratory system starts to develop early in fetal life. The primitive gut forms during the 4th week and is divided into three parts: foregut, midgut, and hindgut. The laryngotracheal tube (the forerunner of the larynx, trachea, and lower respiratory tract), esophagus, stomach, duodenum, and biliary apparatus are some of the derivatives of the foregut. Incomplete division of the foregut into the trachea and esophagus may result in tracheoesophageal fistula, the congenital deformity usually associated with esophageal atresia.[1]

Lung development takes place in four stages:

1. The pseudoglandular period is between 5 and 17 weeks. The major parts of the lung develop during this period, except for those involved with gas exchange. Respiration is not possible during this period.[1]

2. The canalicular period is from 16 to 25 weeks. The bronchi and bronchioles become larger, and the primitive alveolar ducts begin to develop. Lung tissue becomes highly vascular, and respiration is possible during this period.[1]

3. The terminal sac period is from 24 weeks through birth. The alveoli ducts give rise to the terminal sacs and surrounding capillaries. Sufficient alveoli and pulmonary vasculature have developed enough at 26 to 28 weeks for the survival of a premature infant.[1]

4. The alveolar period is from the late fetal period through 8 years of age. The number of bronchioles increases and primitive alveoli enlarge, eventually becoming mature alveoli.[1] From $\frac{1}{8}$ to $\frac{1}{6}$ of the number of alveoli in adults are present in newborn infants. Thus, on chest radiographs of newborn infants, the lungs are denser than those of adults.[1] The contrast seen in adult chest radiographs between the lungs and the surrounding soft tissues is therefore less marked in infants.

At 23 to 24 weeks the alveolar epithelial cells secrete a substance called surfactant. This substance decreases the surface tension at the interface between the air and alveolar surface, maintaining patency of the alveoli and preventing collapse of the lung.[1] When babies are born prematurely, there may be a deficiency of surfactant, resulting in a condition called hyaline membrane disease or respiratory distress syndrome. This condition is the primary cause of respiratory difficulties in newborn infants.

The respiratory system develops so that it is capable of functioning at (term) birth. As a baby is born, the chest is squeezed as it passes through the vagina, forcing the fluid from the lungs. Respiration takes place when sufficient alveoli are present, the alveolo-capillary membrane is thin enough for gas exchange, and an adequate amount of surfactant is present.[1] Growth in the lungs after birth results mainly from an increase in the number of respiratory bronchioles and alveoli, and new alveoli form for at least 8 years after birth.[1]

RADIOGRAPHIC TECHNIQUE

A chest x-ray is the most frequently requested and most poorly performed examination in children. Infants and toddlers are difficult to immobilize and cannot voluntarily suspend respiration; even with short exposure times, the film is frequently exposed during expiration. Centering is often too low because radiographers, more familiar with adult chest radiography, do not take into consideration the shape of the thoracic cavity in infants, which is wider than it is long, and the resultant film tends to have a lordotic appearance. Exposure techniques can vary widely because automatic timing devices do not work well with very young children.

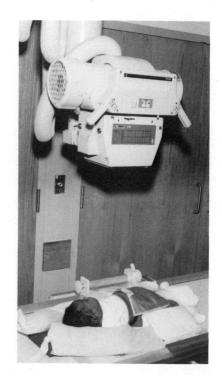

Figure 2–1

A 3-month-old infant positioned for a supine anteroposterior chest radiograph, 40-inch SID.

It is easier to position and immobilize infants and toddlers lying down rather than sitting. A supine anteroposterior projection (Fig. 2–1) and a lateral projection with a horizontal beam are commonly recommended techniques for this age group (see Chapter 10). The lateral is more likely to be a true lateral and will also demonstrate free air or fluid levels. At a distance of 40 inches from source to tabletop (SID), heart magnification is minimal, and the 72-inch SID recommended for older patients is not needed.

A small chest stand attached to the end of the x-ray table or a chest unit specifically designed for preschoolers is helpful for children who can sit with minimal support (Fig. 2–2). Most older children will stand at an upright chest holder by the age of 6 or 7 and with practice will be able to hold their breath on inspiration.

A variety of commercial immobilization devices are available for use with infants and young children. The one we at Children's Hospital have found to be the most effective for toddlers and preschoolers is the Pigg-O-Stat (see Chapter 10). Made of plexiglass, it looks and handles like a straitjacket. Once a child is immobilized in the device, routine views of the chest can be taken quickly and easily. It is important to explain to parents how this device is to be used to avoid being sued for assault and battery—a serious concern, as some parents object to this type of restraint.

One radiographic problem is that the plexiglass that encircles and immobilizes the patient produces linear artifacts on the film. Many radiologists find these confusing, particularly when a pneumothorax is involved. Another concern raised by a radiologist at Children's Hospital is that the device may restrain a child from taking in a deep breath, and the films are not always taken on good inspiration. However, obtaining chest films on inspiration is always problematic in young children. This immobilization device is not suitable for the seriously ill or postoperative patient.

Clothing artifacts are a problem when radiographing small children. The kilovoltage used is not high enough to "burn out" creases or folds, particularly in flame-resistant or unlaundered material. Although care must be taken not to let infants get cold, it

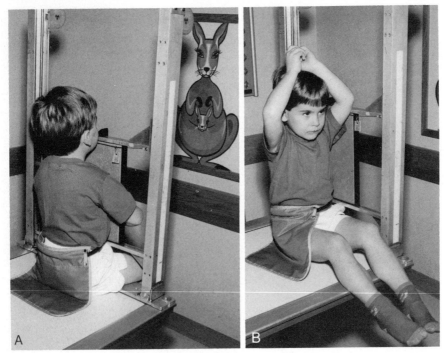

Figure 2–2
A 5-year-old child sitting at a chest stand attached to the x-ray table. **A**, Posteroanterior chest position, 72-inch SID. **B**, Lateral chest position, 72-inch SID.

is better to have them undressed to the waist and the cassette covered by a flat, uncreased sheet. Unfortunately, even though x-ray gowns come in a variety of sizes, they rarely fit children. Plain cotton underpants and t-shirts are the most practical cover-ups. If the hospital does not supply them, suggest to parents that their children wear them to the radiology department. T-shirts or shorts with decals, screen printing, and other decorative designs are not recommended. Hair, particularly braids, can also cause artifacts and cast confusing shadows over the lung fields.

A chest radiograph is a relatively simple, painless examination, but a toddler or preschooler will not think so and needs to be prepared and reassured just as for more complex procedures. Many of us try to reassure children by explaining that they are about to have a "picture taken," the same as having a photograph taken with a camera. This analogy is useful; however, even a small child knows that a big x-ray machine is not the same as a camera at home and will be frightened by the size and loud noises. Simple explanations and constant reassurance will help the examination go more smoothly.

Many chest radiographs are requested as "portable" for inpatient infants. A good mobile machine capable of short exposure times ($\frac{1}{120}$ second or less) should be assigned to a neonatal intensive care unit (NICU). There is a tendency for some radiology departments to allot an old mobile unit to a newborn nursery. The assumption is that the higher generating capacity of newer equipment is not needed to obtain good radiographs on small patients. This is a mistake. Exposure times are too long for patients whose cardiac and respiratory rates are almost always faster than that of adults. The resultant radiographs have a blurred cardiac outline and, in many instances, show respiratory motion.

Collimation should be precise and confined to the thoracic cavity to avoid gonadal exposure. The ovaries tend to be higher in the pelvic cavity in children than in adults, and small half-shields, stocked in different sizes, should be used to absorb fall-off scatter from the edge of the primary beam. Shielding should not be used in lieu of good collimation.

> **Technical Considerations**: A 400-speed screen/film system is recommended for pediatric chest radiography. This combination seems to give the best resolution for the lowest radiation dose. The Department of Radiology at Children's Hospital has experimented with a 600-speed system, but pulmonary detail was less than adequate in radiographs of neonates and infants due to the increase in quantum mottle.

COMMON DISEASES AND CONDITIONS

NEONATES

Respiratory Distress Syndrome

Respiratory distress syndrome and hyaline membrane disease are interchangeable terms for a condition seen in premature infants. The condition is due to immaturity of development and a deficiency of surfactant. The lungs on a radiograph have a ground-glass appearance (Fig. 2–3). A pneumothorax may also be present. These infants are radiographed in their isolettes in the NICU.

With specialized medical and technical support now available, the survival rate for tiny, premature infants is higher. There are 10 to 15 neonates per year at Children's Hospital weighing only 500 to 600 g. Hospitals with birthing facilities may see more. Various tubes and wires measure and monitor every heartbeat, breath, and fluid intake and output of these infants.

Umbilical artery catheters measure oxygen saturation, and umbilical vein and/or peripheral intravenous catheters are used to deliver fluids and medications. There may be a percutaneous or surgically placed central venous line. An endotracheal tube through the nose or the mouth, depending on patient size, is used for suction and mechanical ventilation. Electrocardiograph (EKG) leads on the chest measure cardiac rate and rhythm.

A chest radiograph of a neonate may be taken not only to evaluate the lung fields and heart, but also to check endotracheal tube placement. The position of this tube is critical to within a few millimeters. It should be located above the bifurcation and at or below the thoracic inlet (Fig. 2–4).

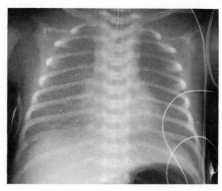

Figure 2–3
A portable anteroposterior chest radiograph showing diffuse ground-glass configuration of the lungs, indicative of hyaline membrane disease. The endotracheal tube is ideally situated 1 cm above the carina.

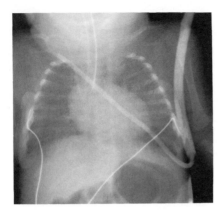

Figure 2–4
Portable anteroposterior chest radiograph of a premature baby weighing less than 1000 g. Mild hyaline membrane disease is present; the heart is slightly enlarged. Note the low endotracheal tube straddling the carina. The electrocardiograph wires and outer portion of the central venous line are lying across the patient.

External tubing and catheters should be moved to the side of the chest and the EKG wires unhooked just before taking the radiograph. Some nurses get understandably anxious at this request, but once the cassette and x-ray tube are in place, the leads can be taken off, the exposure made, and the leads quickly replaced. The less hardware superimposed on the chest, the better for the radiologist reading the film.

> **Routine Projections:** Anteroposterior supine, horizontal ray lateral, and right or left lateral decubitus views on request.

Isolettes in NICU

Radiographers should be familiar with the different types of isolettes used in a newborn nursery or NICU. Two basic types of beds are described here. One is a closed isolette with hand access through portholes (Fig. 2–5). A flow of warm air maintains the inside temperature. Newer models are double walled to help prevent heat loss. The other type is an "open warmer," which has a radiant heater above an open flat bed (Fig. 2–6). In both of these beds, a temperature probe attached to the baby leads to a thermostat that maintains and regulates heat to the neonates. The bed used depends on gestational age, the day of life and the degree of instability.

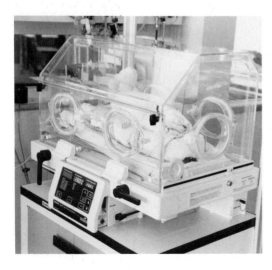

Figure 2–5
Closed isolette with portholes.

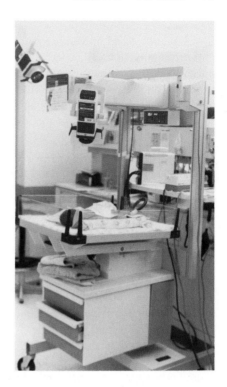

Figure 2-6
Open-bed isolette with overhead warmer that can be moved back to accommodate the x-ray tube.

According to the nurse manager at Children's Hospital, the closed isolettes are preferred for very small babies because they are at high risk and are very sensitive to noise, light, and movement. On the other hand, if an infant is unstable, the open bed allows easier access for placing lines or if the situation suddenly worsens and an "emergency code" is called.

It is essential to keep these babies warm because their body temperatures fall very quickly. Neonates lose a great deal of heat through their skin, particularly the scalp. The skin covers a large area relative to their size, and body temperature can drop by 1°F very quickly. Taking one of these babies out of a warm isolette is analagous to sending an older child or adult outside without a coat on a cold winter day.

Teamwork between the nurse and the radiographer is essential to obtain good diagnostic radiographs of these infants. The radiographer should check the views needed, move the mobile x-ray machine into place, set the technique, cover the cassette, and then position the patient. The heater can be pushed out of the way over the open bed. The closed isolettes usually open from the side and the bed tray slides out. The infant's head, neck, and chest must be straight and collimation precise. Although gonadal protection is recommended, it may be difficult to position on tiny infants. The physicist at Children's Hospital notes that if the chest skin entrance dose for a neonate is 2 mrad (20 μGy), then gonadal dose is estimated at 0.01 mrad (0.1 μGy).[2] This dose assumes a technique of 60 kVp, 0.8 mAs, at 40 inches SID.

INFANTS

Pulmonary Infections

Pulmonary infections in infants 1 to 2 years of age are frequently related to seasonal viral conditions such as pneumonia, parainfluenza types I, II, and III, adenovirus, and respiratory syncytial virus, a highly contagious disease.[3] The virus is shed copiously for days after the onset of the illness, and hospitalized patients must be confined and placed on contact precautions. This disease may cause mild cold symptoms in adults, but it can be lethal for some infants. It is important when radiographing these children to follow strict contact precautions to avoid passing the disease from one patient to another. Viral pneumonia is frequently bilateral with associated hyperinflation and air-trapping.[3] Bronchiolitis is often considered to be a precursor to asthma and is common in children under the age of 1 year[4] (Fig. 2–7).

> **Routine Projections:** Anteroposterior supine and horizontal ray lateral.

Croup and Epiglottitis

Upper respiratory infections in children frequently involve the trachea and the larynx. The larynx of infants differs from the adult larynx in ways other than size. The larynx of infants is relatively high, at the level of the third or fourth cervical vertebra. The epiglottis is narrower, omega-shaped, and more vertical. The subglottic region formed by the relatively immobile cricoid cartilage is the narrowest part of the upper airway. Relatively mild pathologic changes, either congenital or acquired, can result in critical narrowing of the airway.[5]

Children with upper respiratory infections are frequently brought to an emergency room and require immediate radiographs, not only of the chest, but also of the upper airway. Croup and epiglottitis are common causes of breathing difficulties and can lead to dangerous complications in young children.

Croup (laryngotracheobronchitis) may be caused by one of the parainfluenza viruses or by respiratory syncytial virus.[3] The peak incidence is from ages 6 months to 3 years.[3] Onset lasts a few days, and the disease tends to be seasonal, occurring in the winter months. The airway is infected and inflamed, with subglottal tracheal narrowing owing to edema. A harsh barking cough and stridor are present. On the anteroposterior projection, the upper airway shows a steeple-like configuration (Fig. 2–8A). A narrowing of the subglottic portion of the trachea below the level on the larynx can be seen on the lateral projection (Fig. 2–8B).

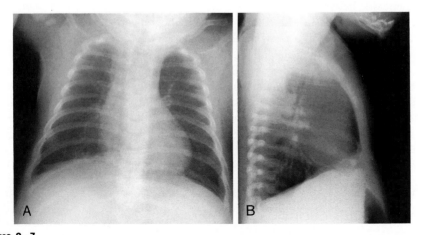

Figure 2–7
A, Supine anteroposterior and **B,** lateral chest radiographs showing diffuse air-trapping and marked flattening of the diaphragm, indicative of bronchiolitis. (The lateral view was taken with a horizontal beam.)

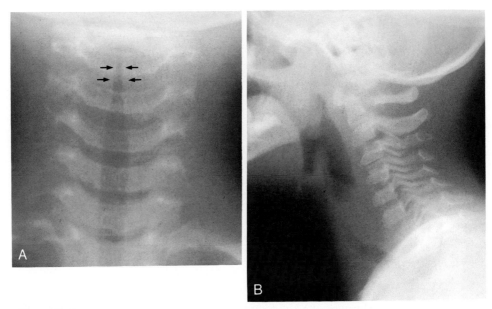

Figure 2–8
A, Anteroposterior radiograph of the neck showing the typical steeple-like configuration of the trachea *(arrows)* seen in patients with croup. *B*, Lateral neck radiograph showing the narrowed infraglottic larynx seen in patients with croup.

Epiglottitis is less common but can be more dangerous. It is a bacterial infection usually due to *Hemophilus influenzae*, with an abrupt onset of symptoms.[3] These patients have great difficulty breathing as the airway is narrowed by the enlarged, swollen epiglottis. Peak incidence is from ages 3 to 6 years.[3] Typically, when patients arrive in the radiology department, they are extremely anxious and tend to lean forward with the neck extended and chest retracted as they try to breathe.

These patients are extremely ill and must always be accompanied by a nurse and a physician to the radiology department. They should be radiographed immediately and in the erect position, as breathing difficulties increase and complete obstruction could occur when the patient is lying down.

Routine Projections: Anteroposterior and lateral chest, anteroposterior and lateral of the upper airway, erect.

Congenital Heart Disease

Congenital heart disease may be initially evaluated by chest radiographs. Heart disease is one of the leading causes of death in infants and children. Congenital cardiac lesions account for approximately 90% of fatalities from heart disease.[4] Radiographic manifestations of congenital heart disease are cardiomegaly, diffuse haziness of the vascular structures, hyperinflation, thymic atrophy, and minor pleural fluid[4] (Fig. 2–9). The thymus gland, normally quite large in young children, spreads out from the mediastinum, which can make it difficult to assess cardiac size radiographically.

Cardiac anomalies are too many and varied to describe here; however, some abbreviations of commonly used terms are listed at the end of this chapter.

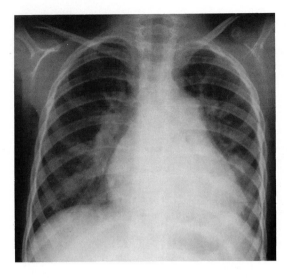

Figure 2–9
Anteroposterior chest radiograph of a 3-year-old child showing cardiomegaly (enlarged heart), a dilated pulmonary artery, and increased pulmonary blood flow.

Routine Projections: Supine anteroposterior and horizontal ray lateral.

Aspirated Foreign Body

Aspiration of a foreign body in the lungs occurs frequently in young children. The sudden onset of a cough without fever suggests aspiration of a foreign object. Aspiration of a foreign body must always be considered in a child under age 3.[3] Children ranging in age from 9 to 16 years aspirate foreign bodies, but peak incidence occurs in children 1 to 2 years of age.[3] Foreign bodies are more common in the right lung than the left because the right bronchus is more in line with the trachea.

Young children test the world around them by putting objects in their mouths. Because the act of aspiration is rarely observed, they should be assumed at risk if they have been given or have found small toys or food items such as peanuts or hard candy.

Radiologic findings include hyperinflation, atelectasis (localized collapse), consolidation, and air-trapping. Normally, the thorax increases in size cross-sectionally on inspiration and decreases on expiration. Air-trapping occurs when the object acts like a valve, allowing air to be inspired but not expired (Fig. 2–10). Because patients in this age group are not able to cooperate with inspiratory and expiratory films, right and left lateral decubitus views are recommended to demonstrate air-trapping on the affected side (Fig. 2–11A). The hyperinflated lung will not deflate when the patient is lying on the affected side (Fig. 2–11B). Fluoroscopy may be an alternative to the decubitus films.

Routine Projections: Anteroposterior supine, horizontal ray lateral, and right and left lateral decubiti.

PRESCHOOL CHILDREN, SCHOOL-AGE CHILDREN, AND ADOLESCENTS

All children are at risk of contracting infectious diseases; thus pneumonia, bronchitis, and influenza are as common in these age groups as in infants, although some

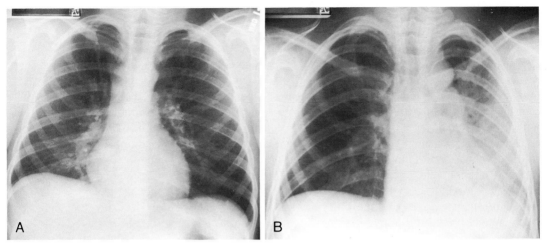

Figure 2–10

This young child aspirated a small plastic Lego building block. **A**, Posteroanterior chest radiograph taken on inspiration. **B**, Posteroanterior chest radiograph taken on expiration showing air-trapping with only moderate deflation of the affected right lung. The Lego, which is not seen in the radiograph owing to its radiolucency, was found in the right main stem bronchus.

diseases may be more prevalent at certain ages than at others. Preschoolers are more susceptible to viral pneumonia, whereas bacterial pneumonia due to pneumococcus, streptococcus, or staphylococcus are more common in older children.[3] Foreign bodies are also found in the lungs of children in these age groups, but older children are more likely to cooperate with obtaining inspiratory and expiratory radiographs to show air-trapping.

Chest radiographs of children in these age groups may be taken erect at a 72-inch SID, either sitting or standing.

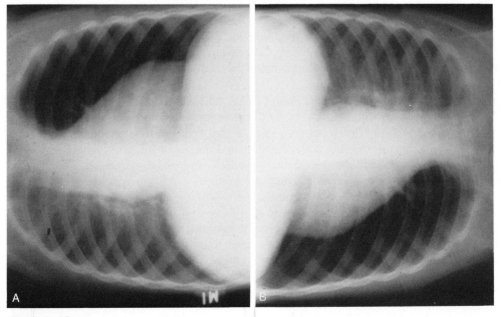

Figure 2–11

Decubitus radiographs of a patient with an aspirated foreign body. **A**, Right lateral decubitus chest radiograph shows normal deflation of the right lung. **B**, Left lateral decubitus radiograph showing nondeflation of the left lung, consistent with air-trapping on that side. (Courtesy of John A. Kirkpatrick, Jr., MD.)

Tuberculosis

Tuberculosis is being diagnosed increasingly in the United States, probably because many of the more recent immigrants are from countries whose health care is substandard and tuberculosis is common. Over 23,000 new cases per year in the United States are now diagnosed, and the number is rising.[4] Of new childhood infections, 40% occur in children from birth to 4 years of age. A significant number of new patients is found in the immunosuppressed population, particularly in the group with AIDS.[4]

Fortunately, if a child is asymptomatic, there is little danger of spread to others. Children produce little sputum; thus, the spread of tuberculosis from child to child is rare; most often a child is infected by the sputum of an adult caretaker.[4] If a child is coughing and producing sputum, contact and respiratory precautions should be performed with gown, gloves, and mask.

Symptoms may be minimal with miliary tuberculosis, with chest radiographs showing multiple nodular opacities throughout the lung fields. Hilar adenopathy and pleural effusion may be present in acutely ill patients.[4]

Routine Projections: Posteroanterior and lateral.

Cystic Fibrosis

A genetic disease, cystic fibrosis is a dysfunction of the exocrine glands. The excessive secretions produced by these glands in this disease create obstruction of the airways. It is most common in Caucasians and uncommon in Blacks and Asians.[4]

In infants, chest radiographs may be normal, and initially meconium ileus is the presenting diagnosis. Symptoms in early childhood include failure to thrive, weight loss, fatigue, malabsorption syndrome, and recurrent pulmonary infections.[4] The diagnosis is confirmed by a positive sweat test.

The viscous mucus accumulates in the airways, causing obstruction and increasing respiratory difficulties (Fig. 2–12). Chest symptoms include recurrent pulmonary infections, cough, upper lobe atelectasis, and pulmonary arterial hypertension. In the 1950's, most affected children died before age 10. Today with aggressive respiratory therapy and antibiotics, many affected individuals live into their 20's and 30's, and even into their 40's and 50's.

As the disease progresses, the child requires frequent hospitalizations for recurrent infections. Standard therapy includes intravenous antibiotics, pulmonary physical therapy, and nutritional support.[6] Progressive mucus plugging of the airways, hyperinflated lungs, flattened diaphragms, bowing of the sternum, and thoracic kyphosis occur (Fig. 2–13). Complications include pneumothorax, pulmonary arterial hypertension, and rupture of the bronchial arteries, with bleeding and hemoptysis.[6] These patients often require bronchial artery occlusion and embolization, and eventually they become candidates for heart and lung transplantations.

A strong emotional support system is essential to help these patients deal with this chronic illness. Frequent trips to the hospital take them away from school, family, and friends, and respiratory difficulties limit their social activities. Depending on the severity and the course of the disease, cystic fibrosis develops into one of the foremost debilitating illnesses of adolescence, and radiographers need to understand the problems facing these teenagers.

Routine Projections: Posteroanterior and lateral.

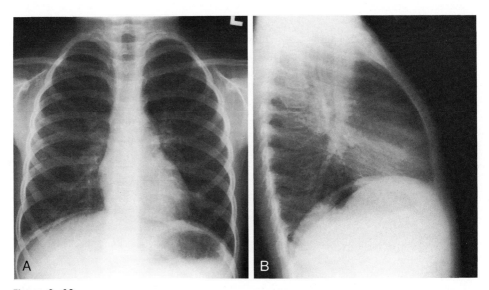

Figure 2–12
A, Posteroanterior and **B**, lateral chest radiographs of an 8-year-old child showing diffuse bronchial wall thickening and cystic nodular changes consistent with cystic fibrosis.

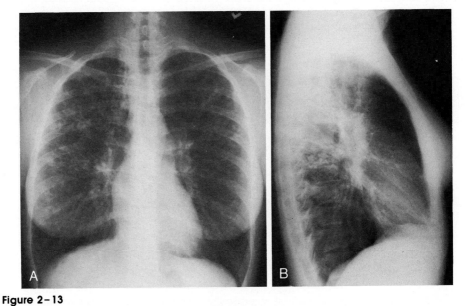

Figure 2–13
A, Posteroanterior and **B**, lateral chest radiographs of a 17-year-old with cystic fibrosis. Diffuse bronchial wall thickening, cystic nodular changes, and some air-trapping are present; the diaphragm is slightly flattened. The lateral projection shows slight thoracic kyphosis and bowing of the sternum. Note streaking on the right side of the neck on the posteroanterior projection from hair draped over the shoulder.

Bronchitis

Bronchitis is an inflammation of the airways that generally occurs secondary to a viral upper respiratory infection. It is a common respiratory ailment of childhood and may also occur in conjunction with asthma or cystic fibrosis. Onset is gradual as the infection spreads to the trachea and bronchi, with a cough appearing after 3 to 4 days.[6] Chest radiographs may appear normal, or peribronchial thickening may be present.[6]

Routine Projections: Posteroanterior and lateral.

Asthma

Asthma, a disorder of the tracheobronchial tree, is characterized by mild to severe narrowing of the airways. Bronchiolitis (inflammation of the bronchioles) is one of the major causes of hospital admission in infants under 1 year and may be a precursor to asthma. In most children, asthma develops before age 8, and in perhaps half of these before age 3.[6] The clinical sign is wheezing—an expiratory sound made through partially obstructed, narrowed airways. Radiographically, the lungs are hyperinflated, the diaphragms flattened, and the bronchial markings increased[6] (Fig. 2–14).

Certain environmental factors tend to promote airway hypersensitivity and precipitate asthma. Attacks are episodic and usually occur after exposure to animals, dust, molds, pollen, and changes in temperature and weather. Status asthmaticus (acute severe asthma) is life-threatening and requires immediate hospitalization.

Routine Projections: Posteroanterior and lateral.

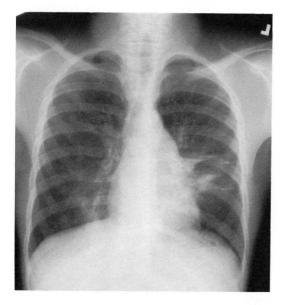

Figure 2–14

Posteroanterior chest radiograph showing multifocal atelectasis (localized collapse), which is more pronounced in the left lung. The diaphragm is flattened, and findings are consistent with chronic asthma.

COMMON CARDIAC ABBREVIATIONS

ASD	Atrial septal defect
BP	Blood pressure
CE	Cardiac enlargement
DM	Diastolic murmur
HLHS	Hypoplastic left heart syndrome
LVH	Left ventricular hypertrophy
MS	Mitral stenosis
M	Murmur
PA	Pulmonary atresia
PBF	Pulmonary blood flow
PS	Pulmonary stenosis
PDA	Patent ductus arteriosus
TGA	Transposition of great arteries
TGV	Transposition of great vessels
TOF	Tetralogy of Fallot
VSD	Ventricular septal defect

REFERENCES

1. Moore, K.L., The Developing Human, W.B. Saunders Company, Philadelphia, 1988
2. Bureau of Radiological Health, Handbook of Selected Organ Doses for Projections Common in Pediatric Radiology, U.S. Department of Health, Education and Welfare, Rockville, MD, May, 1979
3. Hedland, G.L., Kirks, D.R., Respiratory system, in Practical Pediatric Imaging: Diagnostic Radiology of Infants and Children, 2nd ed., pp. 514–707, D. Kirks, ed., Little, Brown & Company, Boston, 1991
4. Silverman, F.N., Kuhn, J.P., Caffey's Pediatric X-ray Diagnosis, 9th ed., Vol. 1, C.V. Mosby Company, St. Louis, 1993
5. Kushner, D.C., Harris, G.B.C., Obstructing Lesions of the Larynx and Trachea in Infants and Children, The Radiological Clinics of North America, W.B. Saunders Company, Philadelphia, 1978
6. Chernick, V., Kendig, E.L., Kendig's Disorders of the Respiratory Tract in Children, W.B. Saunders Company, Philadelphia, 1990

Chapter 3

The Abdomen

DEVELOPMENT OF THE DIGESTIVE TRACT

In the developing embryo, the primitive digestive tract is a tube that, for descriptive purposes, consists of three parts: the foregut, midgut, and hindgut. The foregut gives rise to the pharynx, lower respiratory system, esophagus, stomach, first and second parts of the duodenum, liver, pancreas, and biliary apparatus. The trachea and esophagus have a common origin; therefore, incomplete partitioning may result in, for example, esophageal atresia (an esophagus with a blind end) with or without tracheoesophageal fistulae.[1]

The midgut gives rise to the distal part of the duodenum, jejunum, ileum, cecum, appendix, and ascending colon to the midtransverse colon. The midgut forms a U-shaped loop that herniates into the umbilical cord during the 6th week of embryonic development because of lack of space in the abdominal cavity. While it is in the umbilical cord it rotates counterclockwise through 90 degrees. During the 10th week, the intestines return to the abdomen, rotating another 180 degrees.[1] The remainder of the transverse colon, the descending and sigmoid colons, the rectum, and most of the anal canal develop from the hindgut.

Alimentary tract anomalies seen in the newborn and infant are the result of abnormal embryonic development. The rotation and fixation of the intestine as it returns from the umbilical sac into the abdominal cavity normally results in the mesentery's being fixed in the left upper quadrant by the ligament of Treitz, with the other end in the right iliac fossa.[1]

At birth, with the colon in its normal position, the large bowel forms a frame around the small bowel. Nonrotation occurs when the midgut does not rotate as it returns to the abdomen, so that the small bowel lies to the right side and the large bowel to the left side of the abdomen. Malrotation or incomplete rotation results in a condition that is between nonrotation and normal.

If normal rotation and fixation of the bowel does not take place, the small bowel can twist on itself. This causes an obstruction of the lumen and, in some cases, strangulation of the superior mesenteric artery and vein, with subsequent infarction. Nonrotation may be an incidental finding in older children, but malrotation with volvulus (twisting of the intestine) usually is present in neonates and infants.

Malformation of the hindgut accounts for Hirschsprung disease, which, because of the absence of autonomic ganglion cells, commonly causes a narrowing at the sigmoid-rectal junction. Other abnormalities include imperforate anus and anorectal fistulae.

At birth, the abdomen and thorax in the infant are equal in circumference. Musculature is poorly developed, the abdomen is prominent, the pelvis is small, and the pelvic viscera are higher than in older children. On plain radiographs of infants and young children it is difficult to differentiate between the small and large bowels. The gas-filled loops tend to look the same, whereas in adults the haustra of the large bowel are clearly visible. Thus, if a horizontal loop of bowel follows the greater curvature of the stomach, it is most likely transverse colon; if a vertical loop of gut is visible in the pelvis, it is probably rectum.

Infants breathe abdominally, and it is difficult to keep a gonadal shield in place on the protruding, wobbly abdomen of such young patients. Because there is little intrinsic fat, the abdominal organs (such as the kidneys) are not as well defined on a plain radiograph of the abdomen as they are in adults. As a child grows, stands, and walks, the vertebral curves develop, muscles strengthen, and the abdomen flattens, although the potbellied stance of some children may persist until age 11.

RADIOGRAPHIC TECHNIQUE

Plain radiographs of the abdomen are always taken before gastrointestinal or genitourinary studies for evaluation of soft tissues before the introduction of barium or iodine contrast media. Plain radiographs, particularly of the acute abdomen in children, provide valuable diagnostic information to the radiologist.

Normal babies cry and swallow air. It is normal to see air throughout the gastrointestinal tract, but it should be evenly distributed. Plain radiographs of the abdomen for infants and children should be considered contrast studies of the intestine using air. The supine radiograph should be supplemented with a prone view as well as other views to distribute the gas throughout the colon and bowel.[2] Kirks and Caron also recommend the following acute abdomen series: anteroposterior supine, posteroanterior prone, and a left lateral or supine horizontal ray lateral.[2]

The supine preliminary radiograph should include the abdomen from the diaphragm to the pubic symphysis (Fig. 3–1). Overcollimation in neonates and infants should be avoided, because it is important to include the outer edges of the abdomen. Subtle changes that affect the soft-tissue outlines in younger children are usually "burned out" at the higher kilovoltages used for larger, older patients (and adults).

> **Technical Considerations:** A 400-speed screen/film system is recommended for radiography of the abdomen.

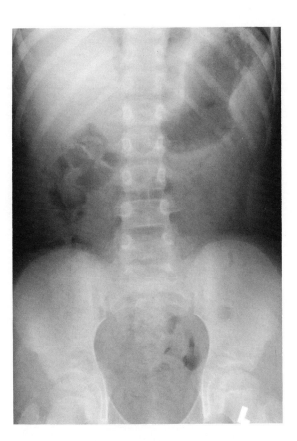

Figure 3–1

Normal supine anteroposterior radiograph of the abdomen of an 8-year-old girl. Note spina bifida occulta at S1. This may close later.

COMMON DISEASES AND CONDITIONS

NEONATES

Atresias

In certain situations, a radiograph that includes both the chest and abdomen (sometimes called a "babygram") may be requested as a portable examination for a neonate. Technically it is easy to do because the procedure does not require a grid.

Unless a baby is premature and weighs less than 1000 g, it is preferable to radiograph the chest and abdomen separately when the abdomen and chest are of similar size and the lungs are not well aerated. Many radiologists feel that the chest appears too dark and the abdomen too light when both are included in one radiograph, thus compromising the diagnostic value of the examination.

Many congenital abnormalities of the gastrointestinal tract are evident soon after birth. For example, esophageal atresia is suspected if the neonate is choking and spitting as secretions spill into the hypopharynx instead of going down the esophagus. This abnormality may be demonstrated on plain radiographs by the air that collects in the blind pouch proximal to the atresia. The lateral view is most useful, because gas in the cigar-shaped esophageal pouch will push against the posterior aspect of the trachea, causing it to narrow and bow anteriorly (Fig. 3–2).

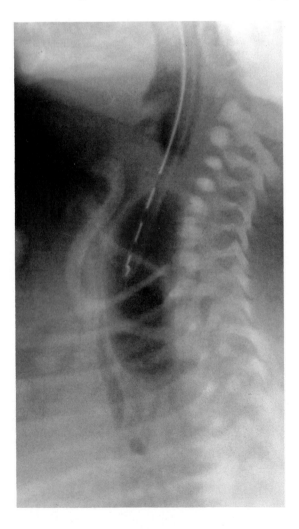

Figure 3–2

Lateral radiograph of the neck showing the esophageal pouch outlined by air. The trachea is narrowed and bowed anteriorly.

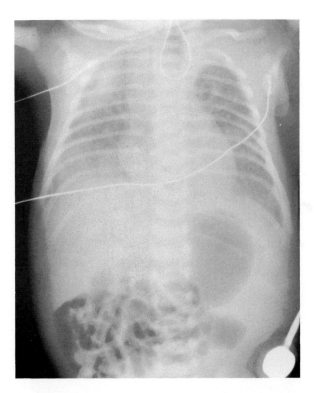

Figure 3-3
Anteroposterior radiograph showing a catheter coiled in the esophagus at the level of the upper pouch of the atresia. Air is seen in the bowel, indicating a tracheoesophageal fistula. There is diffuse irregular lung disease caused by either reflux of gastric contents or aspiration of secretions from above.

Esophageal atresia may be accompanied by a tracheoesophageal fistula. If communication exists between the lower portion of the esophagus and the gastrointestinal tract (sometimes there is more than one fistula), gas will be present in the stomach and bowel (Fig. 3-3). An abdomen devoid of gas means no fistula is present and therefore there is no communication between the trachea and the gastrointestinal tract (Fig. 3-4).

In duodenal atresia, which most commonly occurs at the level of the second part of the duodenum, a double gas bubble will be present on a plain radiograph of the abdomen. The large bubble is the stomach, and the small bubble is the duodenal bulb.[2] In jejunal atresia, gas will be present in the dilated stomach and loops of proximal small bowel. In both conditions, the abdomen will be devoid of gas beyond the level of the obstruction.

> **Routine Projections:** Anteroposterior and horizontal ray lateral (to confirm the level of the obstruction), and anteroposterior and lateral chest to include the neck (to detect esophageal atresia).

Diaphragmatic Hernia

Diaphragmatic hernias are of various types depending on the congenital abnormality. All such abnormalities result in the herniation of the abdominal contents into the thoracic cavity, mostly on the left side (Fig. 3-5). Respiration may be severely compromised by the gas-filled loops in the thorax. The lung on the side of the hernia is incompletely developed (hypoplastic), and function of the contralateral lung is variably affected.

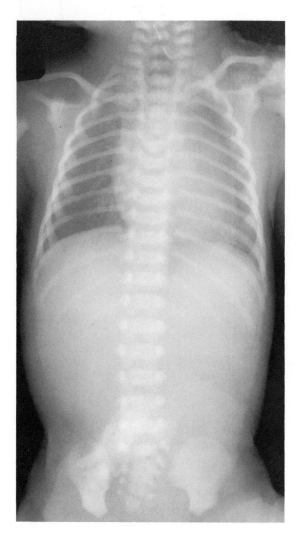

Figure 3–4
No gas is present in the bowel of this patient with esophageal atresia, indicating that no connection exists between the esophagus and the trachea. Note the abnormal sacrum.

Babies with this condition need surgical intervention and may require special life support, such as extracorporeal membrane oxygenation. This mechanically assisted oxygenation of the blood is used before and after surgery.

Routine Projections: Anteroposterior supine and horizontal ray lateral views of the chest and abdomen.

Meconium Plug Syndrome

Meconium plug syndrome is an obstruction of the normal passage of meconium through the left colon either because of a plug of meconium or because of a hypoactive bowel. The abdomen is distended, and loops of small and large bowel are dilated. There may be a soap-bubble appearance in the distribution of gas and fluid in the ascending and transverse colons.

Routine Projections: Anteroposterior supine and horizontal ray lateral.

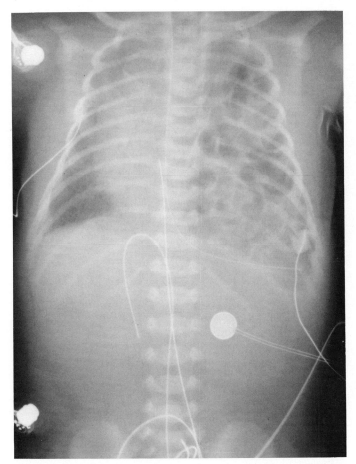

Figure 3–5
Anteroposterior chest radiograph of a newborn showing multiple loops of bowel in the left hemithorax, consistent with a diaphragmatic hernia.

Meconium Ileus

Meconium ileus is peculiar to patients with cystic fibrosis, a genetic disease of the exocrine glands in which both the lungs and intestinal tract produce abnormal amounts of sticky mucus (see Chapter 2). Ten to twenty percent of patients with cystic fibrosis are obstructed at birth by the accumulation of meconium in the distal small bowel, which causes a meconium ileus.[2]

The colon is unused and therefore small in caliber because of the obstruction at the level of the ileum. After birth, a plain radiograph of the abdomen will show a soap-bubble appearance in the right lower quadrant as air, gradually passing into the digestive tract, mixes with the meconium. The small bowel is usually dilated but without air-fluid levels on decubitus or cross-table lateral radiographs.

Routine Projections: Anteroposterior supine and horizontal ray lateral.

Meconium Ileus Equivalent

Older children with cystic fibrosis produce abnormal amounts of mucus, which mixes with feces, causing an obstruction of the terminal ileum and cecum (Fig. 3–6).

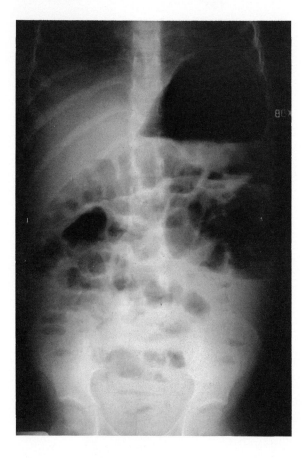

Figure 3–6
Upright anteroposterior radiograph of an abdomen showing multiple air-fluid levels in a patient with cystic fibrosis, indicative of meconium ileus equivalent.

For patients with meconium ileus equivalent (an acquired complication), a meglumine diatrizoate enema rather than a barium enema is sometimes performed, as it clears the adherent stool from the bowel. Meglumine diatrizoate differs from the other iodinated contrast materials in that it contains Tween 80, a wetting agent that acts like a detergent.

Routine Projections: Anteroposterior supine and erect.

Imperforate Anus

Imperforate anus is the failure of the large bowel to terminate properly. There is no anal opening because of abnormal development of the hindgut.[2] Radiographs are taken to try to determine the level of the termination. The radiographic positioning methods suggested in the literature are not always accurate, because the meconium in the distal rectum may mimic obstruction and malformation at a higher level. This inaccuracy is particularly true of the inverted lateral abdomen position, which used to be a popular method of assessing the level of rectal termination.

It is suggested that films not be taken until the baby is 18 to 24 hours old to ensure the presence of sufficient gas in the rectum to demonstrate the level of the lesion and its relationship to the perineum.[2]

Many patients born with anorectal malformations have fistulae that communicate with the genital or urinary tract. In females, fistulae tend to communicate with the genital tract, whereas in males, the communication is with the urinary tract.[2] The extent of these fistulae may be demonstrated under fluoroscopy with a water-soluble contrast medium (Fig. 3–7). Because associated renal and bladder abnormalities are usually present as well, intravenous pyelography or renal ultrasonography and voiding cystourethrography are frequently performed.

Routine Projections: Place a lead marker on the perineum at the dimple where the anal opening would normally be. Anteroposterior supine, posteroanterior prone and prone horizontal ray lateral.

Hirschsprung Disease

The symptoms of Hirschsprung disease — intermittent constipation, distention, and occasionally diarrhea — date from birth, although Hirschsprung disease may not be diagnosed until later in life. Ganglion cells are absent in the distal portion of the large bowel, frequently in the area of the rectosigmoid region, causing a narrowing of the bowel.[2] Rarely, the entire colon may be affected. Feces cannot pass through the narrowed, dysfunctional portion; therefore, they become impacted, and the colon proximal to the narrowing becomes dilated (Fig. 3–8).

Depending on the extent of the disease, plain radiographs of the abdomen may show dilatation of the gastrointestinal tract above the level of the obstruction. Air-fluid levels are commonly visible on an upright view of the abdomen. Preparation by catharsis or cleansing enema may produce a false-negative result. Patients with suspected Hirschsprung disease should not be given laxatives before a barium enema (see preparation for barium enema in Appendix B).

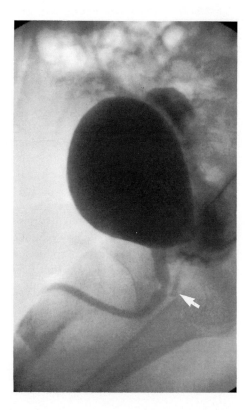

Figure 3–7
Voiding cystourethrogram of a neonate with imperforate anus. *Arrow* points to a fistula between the urethra and rectum.

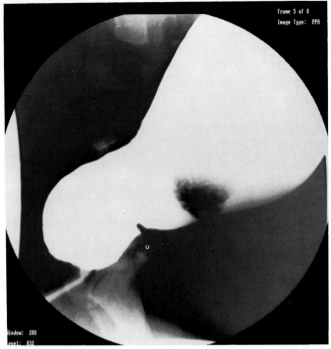

Figure 3-8
Barium outlines the narrowing (transitional zone) between the rectum and the dilated proximal sigmoid colon.

Routine Projections: Anteroposterior supine, posteroanterior prone, prone cross-table lateral, and upright (to show air-fluid levels).

INFANTS AND PRESCHOOL CHILDREN

Pyloric Stenosis

Pyloric stenosis is the most common abdominal condition in infants. Symptoms occur at 2 to 6 weeks of age, with peak incidence at 3 weeks. The infant will have frequent nonbilious vomiting, which may become projectile after feeding.[2] On a plain radiograph of the abdomen, the stomach will be distended and out of proportion with the rest of the gastrointestinal tract because of gas and fluid. A figure-eight configuration is evident. If the greater curvature of the stomach reaches the fourth lumbar vertebra or below, it is probably pathologically distended (Fig. 3-9).

Although radiographs were traditionally followed by a barium study (Fig. 3-10A), ultrasonography has become the imaging modality of choice to measure the length and thickness of the hypertrophied pyloric muscle, which is the cause of the delay in stomach emptying (Fig. 3-10B).

Routine Projection: Anteroposterior supine.

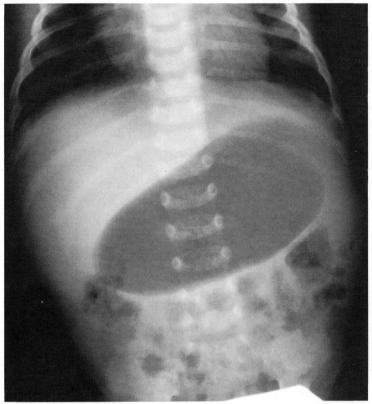

Figure 3–9
Supine anteroposterior radiograph of an abdomen showing gaseous distension of the stomach with little air in the small and large bowel, consistent with pyloric stenosis.

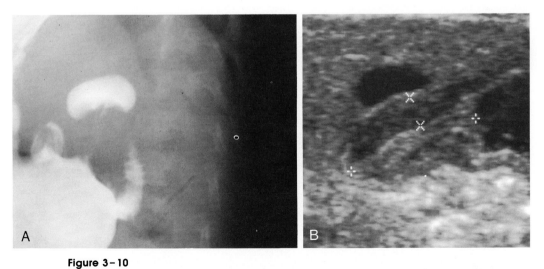

Figure 3–10
A, Barium study showing an elongated and narrowed pyloric canal. *B*, Ultrasound showing elongation of the pyloric canal *(asterisks)* and thickened pyloric muscle *(crosses)*.

Intussusception

In intussusception, the bowel telescopes inside itself, causing an obstruction and severe abdominal pain. A normal plain radiograph of the abdomen does not exclude intussusception, although a soft-tissue mass may be seen in the area of the intussusception. The symptoms are classic: a well child will suddenly bend over, grab his belly, cry with pain, and pass a reddish-black gelatinous material defined as "currant jelly stool."

Children between the ages of 3 months and 2½ years may suddenly develop idiopathic (of unknown origin) intussusception. Some physicians think it follows a viral enteritis. Lymphoid tissue (Peyer's patches) in the gastrointestinal tract is larger in infants and becomes larger after infection. Peyer's patches may act as a lead point in the bowel as it telescopes inside itself, causing an obstruction.[2]

In children under 3 months and over 3 years of age, intussusception may be associated with a lead point such as Meckel's diverticulum. This common congenital abnormality of the small bowel is due to the persistence of the most distal portion of the duct between the yolk sac and the ileum.

Intussusception is reduced hydrostatically under fluoroscopy by a radiologist using air (Fig. 3–11), a water-soluble contrast material, or barium (Fig. 3–12). Perforation is always a risk. Air is considered much less hazardous than barium, even with the possible complication of leakage of fecal material into the peritoneal cavity.

Three to six percent of hydrostatically reduced intussusceptions recur. The most important radiograph is of the supine abdomen, postevacuation after reduction (Fig. 3–13). If contrast did not reflux into the ileum, or if the small bowel is completely devoid of contrast material after evacuation, the intussusception has probably recurred.

It is very important to realize that a child with this condition is in a great deal of pain, and introducing contrast into the bowel will increase the pain. When reduction is successful, the child becomes quiet and often falls asleep.

Routine Projections: Anteroposterior supine, posteroanterior prone, and supine horizontal ray lateral. A child of 2 years or older may stand for an erect radiograph of the abdomen.

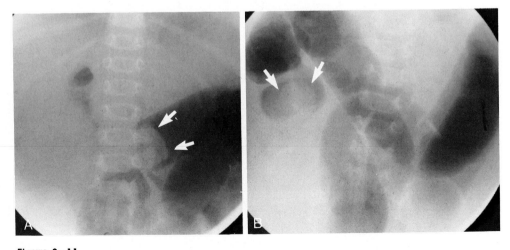

Figure 3–11
Fluoroscopic spot radiographs showing the lead point of intussusception as it is being reduced by an air enema. **A**, The lead point in the transverse colon *(arrows)*. **B**, The lead point in the ascending colon *(arrows)*.

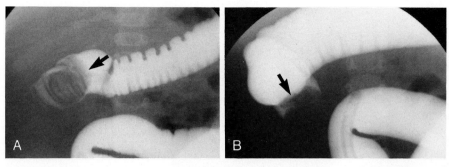

Figure 3–12

Fluoroscopic spot radiographs showing the lead point of intussusception as it is being reduced by a barium enema. **A**, The lead point in transverse colon *(arrow)*. **B**, The lead point in ascending colon *(arrow)*.

Malrotation

Again, a normal plain radiograph of the abdomen does not exclude a particular condition. The patient's medical history is critical because malrotation can be catastrophic for a child. Symptoms include intermittent bilious vomiting. The vomiting may start and stop, then start again as the small bowel twists (volvulus) and then untwists. The child may seem quite well between attacks, and parents may believe the child has recovered from a gastric upset. The yellowish-green vomitus is the clue to the seriousness of the condition.

The cardinal radiographic sign of malrotation is the abnormal placement of the duodenal-jejunal junction (Fig. 3–14). This portion of the intestine, when made opaque by barium, should be visible in the left upper quadrant, behind the stomach, at the level of the ligament of Treitz. Malrotation of the midgut with volvulus may cause infarction of the gut as the small bowel twists around the superior mesenteric artery and vein, cutting off its own blood supply (Fig. 3–15). This condition is life threatening, since

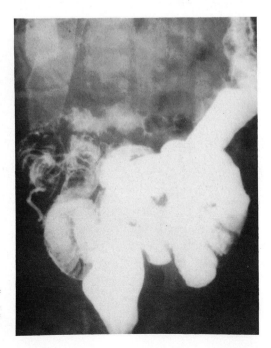

Figure 3–13

Supine anteroposterior radiograph of the abdomen showing barium in the terminal ileum after reduction of intussusception.

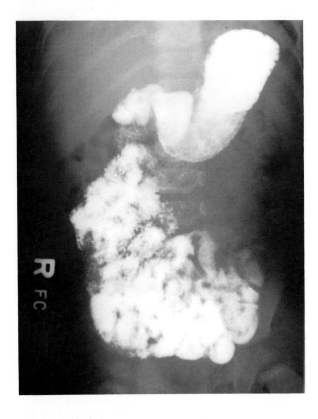

Figure 3–14
Barium study showing the duo-denojejunal junction slightly to the right of the midline and inferior to the normal location.

one cannot live without a small bowel. The evaluation of affected children should be expedited.

Routine Projections: Anteroposterior supine and upright. Older children may stand for an erect radiograph.

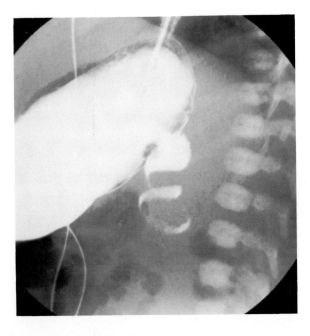

Figure 3–15
Barium study showing malrotation with volvulus.

SCHOOL-AGE CHILDREN AND ADOLESCENTS

Appendicitis

Acute appendicitis is the most frequent condition requiring abdominal surgery in children.[2] The disease is rare in infants and more common in older children. The symptoms are abdominal pain that becomes localized to the right lower quadrant, nausea, vomiting, and fever.

The plain radiograph of the abdomen may be completely normal, but an appendicolith (calcified fecalith) in the right lower quadrant (Fig. 3–16) with the symptoms listed is indicative of appendicitis. Inflammatory changes indicate the possible presence of an obstruction, which will be demonstrated by air-fluid levels on an erect or decubitus view of the abdomen. An abscess may be seen as a soft-tissue mass. Localized edema may obscure the line of the right psoas muscle, although this is not as well defined in younger children. Pain may cause the spine to be pulled toward the left side, creating a temporary, mild scoliosis.

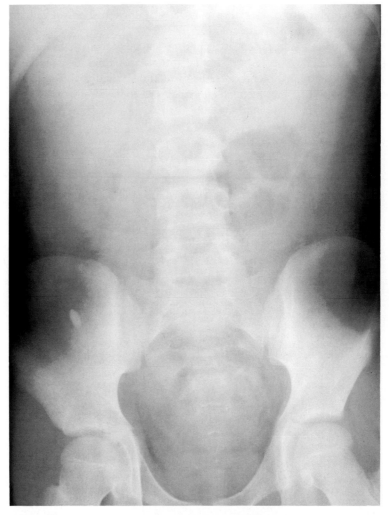

Figure 3–16

Supine anteroposterior radiograph of the abdomen showing a fecalith in the right lower quadrant.

> **Routine Projections:** Anteroposterior supine and erect and/or left lateral decubitus.

Crohn Disease and Ulcerative Colitis

Crohn disease, also commonly known as regional enteritis or granulomatous colitis, can affect both the small and large bowels and is a common inflammatory disease in children. Peak incidence is in young adulthood, but 25% of patients are diagnosed in childhood or adolescence.[3] The disease may be localized to one segment or may involve several segments with normal bowel between them.[3] The terminal ileum is most frequently involved.

Symptoms include diarrhea, abdominal pain, anorexia, abdominal mass, and fistula in ano.[3] Extraintestinal symptoms include failure to thrive, arthritis, sacroiliitis, erythema nodosa, or fever. The lumen of the intestine is narrowed by the fibrotic thickened walls and by spasm, sometimes called the "string sign." The ulcerations give a "cobblestone" appearance, which is typically visible on a barium study[3] (Fig. 3–17). The plain radiograph may be normal or may show a thickened bowel wall and loss of the normal haustral pattern of the colon.

Ulcerative colitis is diagnosed in teenagers but may also present in children as young as 4 years. The symptoms are similar to those of Crohn disease, depending on the severity. As with adults, bloody diarrhea is common, and with the progression of the disease, patients become anemic, anorexic, and underweight and generally feel miserable. It is a debilitating condition, and the diarrhea becomes a social problem.

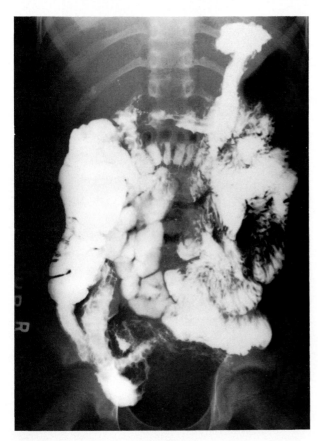

Figure 3–17
Follow-through barium study of the small bowel showing extensive "cobblestone" appearance of the distal ileum in a patient with bowel thickening consistent with Crohn disease.

Patients always face the prospect of toxic megacolon and perforation. A colectomy may be performed to prevent colonic carcinoma,[4] which rarely occurs in children, but patients with ulcerative colitis are at a higher risk later in life.[4]

Routine Projections: Anteroposterior supine and erect (to include the diaphragm for free air when perforation is a possibility).

Constipation

Chronic constipation is one of the most common reasons children are referred for a radiographic examination of the abdomen. Plain radiographs are taken to (1) confirm the presence of stool throughout the colon and (2) determine whether the constipation is functional or due to disease (Fig. 3-18). For example, a child with a delayed diagnosis of Hirschsprung disease would have a history of chronic constipation.

Encopresis (involuntary passage of feces) in an otherwise well child may be due to functional constipation and may be psychosomatic. Plain radiographs, sometimes followed by a barium enema, are taken to rule out underlying disease. If no other problem is detected, these patients are put on a special diet and referred for behavior therapy.

Routine Projection: Anteroposterior supine.

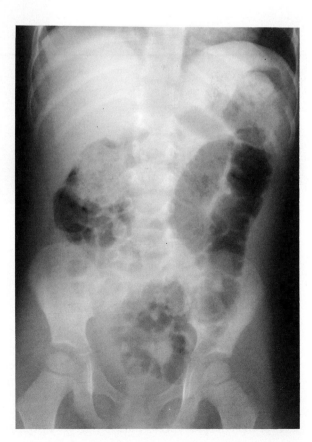

Figure 3-18

Supine anteroposterior radiograph of the abdomen showing gas and impacted feces in a patient with chronic constipation.

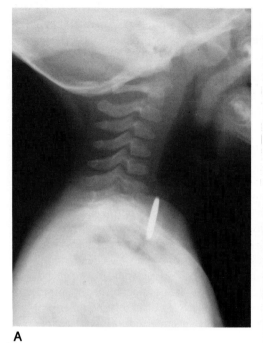

A

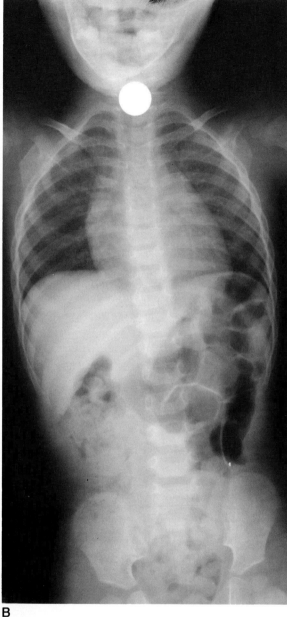

B

Figure 3–19
A, Lateral neck radiograph of an 18-month-old child showing a coin lodged at the level of the cricopharyngeal muscle. *B*, Supine anteroposterior radiograph of the chest and abdomen of the same patient.

Meconium Ileus Equivalent

(See the section on neonates.)

Ingested Foreign Body

Young children, toddlers in particular, typically put inappropriate objects in their mouths. They may either swallow or inhale a foreign object. A swallowed object that is small, round, and without sharp edges (like a small coin) will most likely pass through the digestive tract without complication.

Depending on the age and size of the child, larger objects may get lodged at the level of the cricopharyngeus muscle (Fig. 3–19*A*), the thoracic inlet, the aortic arch, the lower end of the esophagus (as it enters the stomach), or the pyloric sphincter. Once a foreign body has passed through the stomach, it will usually continue all the way through the small and large intestines.

Nonmetallic objects are difficult to see on a radiograph, although it sometimes helps to radiograph a similar object immersed in water to determine its radio-opacity. This does not always work; a piece of plastic may be visible by itself on a radiograph and then be obscured by the shadows of the chest and abdominal tissue. However, this process is worth a try if a similar object is available.

Small straight pins, although metal, can blur with peristalsis, but because they carry the risk of perforation, as do other sharp objects, localization is important. Anteroposterior and lateral projections should be taken to assist in localizing the object.

When radiographing a patient who has ingested a foreign body, it is important to radiograph not only the abdomen but the entire alimentary tract from mouth to anus (Fig. 3–19B). If the abdomen is radiographed before the thorax, there is the risk that the foreign body will have moved from the esophagus to the stomach between exposures and will not be seen on either radiograph.

When a foreign object is swallowed, it may scratch the esophagus, and a distressed patient and parent may think it is lodged there. Radiographs should begin at the lateral neck, followed by the chest, and then the abdomen. Except for the lateral neck, infants fit on one 14-inch by 17-inch film, which precludes overlooking a foreign body between the thorax and the abdomen.

Routine Projections: Lateral neck, anteroposterior and lateral chest, anteroposterior and lateral abdomen.

REFERENCES

1. Moore, Keith L., The Developing Human, W.B. Saunders Company, Philadelphia, 1988
2. Kirks, Donald R., Caron, Kathleen H., Gastrointestinal tract, in Practical Pediatric Imaging: Diagnostic Radiology of Infants and Children, 2nd ed., pp. 708–903, D. Kirks, Ed., Little, Brown & Company, Boston, 1991
3. Silverman, F.N., Kuhn, J.P., Caffey's Pediatric Diagnosis, 9th ed., Vol. 1, C.V. Mosby Company, St. Louis, Vol. 1, 1993
4. Schapiro, R.L., Clinical Radiology of the Pediatric Abdomen and Gastrointestinal Tract, University Park Press, Baltimore, 1976

Chapter 4

The Gastrointestinal Tract

FLUOROSCOPY OF THE GASTROINTESTINAL TRACT

Radiography and fluoroscopy of the gastrointestinal (GI) tract is less complicated in children than in adults. In adults, the shape and position of abdominal organs vary with body size and shape and with muscle tone. In children, there is little variation in the location of the stomach and intestines until puberty. Preparation is minimal, fewer radiographs are taken, and fluoroscopy time is shorter because motility is more rapid, except in certain pathologic conditions. There is a concerted effort to keep radiation doses low.

Many pediatric abnormalities and diseases requiring contrast for further evaluation have been discussed in Chapter 3. A plain radiograph of the abdomen should always be taken to evaluate soft tissues and gas patterns before the introduction of contrast material. If a barium swallow is specifically requested as well as an upper gastrointestinal (UGI) series, a posteroanterior and a lateral view of the chest should also be done.

To better identify abnormal anatomy and pathology, barium, air, or an iodinated contrast material is either swallowed or introduced via catheter into the alimentary tract, and patients are examined under fluoroscopy. Fluoroscopic examinations include a barium swallow for the esophagus, UGI study for the stomach and duodenum, a small-bowel follow-through for the jejunum and ileum, and a barium enema for visualization of the cecum and remainder of the large bowel. The combination, sequence, and type of contrast used is dependent on the patient's age and the clinical diagnosis.

A barium swallow is rarely performed without a UGI study in young children. A UGI study with small-bowel follow-through is a common procedure. A barium enema, with or without air contrast, is used less frequently. Although a double-contrast enema is nearly always a standard procedure with adults, it is rarely performed with children except when used for a diagnosis of polyps as a cause of rectal bleeding. Bowel cancer is rare in children.

PATIENT AND ROOM PREPARATION

The fluoroscopic procedure room should be completely prepared before a patient enters the room. The table should be in the horizontal position and draped with cotton or disposable sheeting. A sheet (12 inches by 24 inches, depending on the width of the table) of 1-mm lead vinyl should be placed on the table and positioned beneath the child's buttocks during a barium swallow and UGI study. This will help protect the child's gonads from scatter radiation when an undercouch fluoroscopic x-ray tube is used. It will also protect the fluoroscopist's hands, although most radiologists wear a lead glove on the right hand.

Radiographic controls, depending on equipment design, should be set for fluoroscopy, regular spot films, a 100-mm camera, videotape, or a digital spot film device for recording images. Depending on the procedure, the appropriate barium, nonionic contrast medium, feeding bottle, nipples, cup, straws, spoons, feeding catheter, and syringe should be laid out and ready to use, along with towels and washcloths to clean up with after the procedure (Fig. 4–1). Oxygen and suction should also be readily available for emergency situations.

The child and parent should be brought into the room before the fluoroscopic procedure starts. The radiologist and radiographer should introduce themselves to the parent and patient. While the radiologist explains the examination to the parent, the radiographer can explain the equipment and how it works to the child. Even very young children benefit from being familiarized with the room and the procedure. The

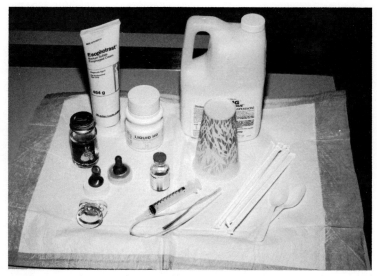

Figure 4-1
Barium, a nonionic contrast medium, a feeding bottle, nipples, a cup, straws, spoons, a feeding catheter, and a syringe used for upper gastrointestinal tract studies.

radiographer should explain how they will drink a "milk shake," and how they can watch it go down into their stomach on the television monitor. Let the parents stay in the room with their child, and — most important to parents — tell them how long it will take, particularly if follow-up radiographs will be taken. This small amount of preparation is worth the time spent in helping to reduce anxiety and creating a positive, supportive environment.

Some radiologists prefer to keep a firm grip on the legs and thus move the patient around manually. Others use an immobilization device such as the octagonal board. The radiographer can feed the child with the help of a parent at the head of the table. Words of encouragement should be given continually until the required amount of barium has gone down. Patients undergoing small-bowel studies can finish their barium while sitting in the waiting room.

UPPER GASTROINTESTINAL TRACT STUDIES

PATIENT PREPARATION

Infants and young children require minimal preparation for UGI studies, and fasting is the main requirement. Length of fasting is determined by age. Three to four hours is adequate for babies, which usually means forgoing the feed immediately prior to the examination (babies can have an early morning feed at 6 a.m. and be ready for a UGI study at 10 a.m.). Children over 1 year of age should go without solids and liquids for 4 to 6 hours. The older the child, the slower the gastric emptying.

Hungry babies cry, and every attempt should be made not to keep a parent and fasting baby waiting for their appointment. One advantage is that a hungry baby takes a bottle of barium easily and does not seem to mind the taste. Older children may refuse to drink the barium and may spit it out even when it is flavored. Persuading a child to drink this milk shake is a challenge for any radiographer.

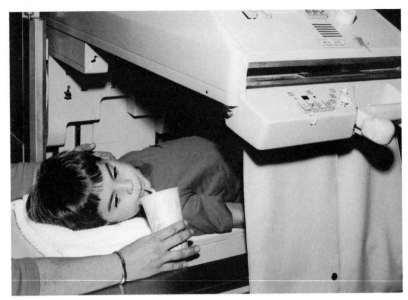

Figure 4–2
A recumbent 5-year-old child sipping barium through a straw during fluoroscopy.

Barium can be sipped from a cup or through a straw (Fig. 4–2), but if a child refuses to drink, the radiographer needs to become creative. While a hungry and thirsty child may find the barium more tolerable, difficulties generally arise when toddlers start to develop likes and dislikes about food.

Our expert radiographer on barium studies advises holding the nose gently but firmly, and when the child's mouth opens, trying to squirt barium into the side of the mouth with a 10-cc syringe. Also, barium paste can be spooned under the palate or onto the tongue. Holding the child under the lower jaw helps prevent spitting it out.

Sometimes we send the parent and child to the waiting room and ask the parent to persuade the child to drink the barium while watching television or reading a story. If the esophagus was not evaluated beforehand, barium paste can be given when the child returns to be fluoroscoped. If all else fails, it may be necessary for the radiologist to pass a nasogastric tube into the child's stomach.

Barium sulfate is the contrast of choice except when there is a question of GI perforation or necrosis. Diatrizoate meglumine and diatrizoate sodium solution, an iodine-based oral contrast medium, is sometimes used as a substitute for barium, but its hyperosmolality causes fluid to be drawn into the bowel, disrupting electrolyte balance. Diatrizoate meglumine and diatrizoate sodium solution can cause peritonitis if it leaks into the peritoneum, and chemical pneumonitis if it is aspirated. It is also extremely bitter to drink, and the taste is hard to disguise. When barium is contraindicated, most radiologists use a nonionic contrast medium because of its low toxicity.

If a radiographic requisition requests a barium swallow, most radiologists will continue fluoroscopy to check the stomach and duodenal loop. It is important to identify the location of the duodenojejunal junction in case of a previously undiagnosed malrotation. Early detection of malrotation before symptoms appear could save a child's life.

Patient Preparation for Barium Swallow and UGI Study

Newborn to 2 years	Nothing by mouth 3 to 4 hours.
Over 2 years	Nothing by mouth for 6 hours.
(See Appendices A and B)	

BARIUM PREPARATION

Liquid barium, 40% weight/weight and 60% weight/volume, may be used or diluted according to a particular manufacturer's instruction. Neonates and infants may require it slightly more dilute. Warm or tepid, rather than cold, water added to powder or barium in suspension at room tempertaure is palatable. Most products are artificially fruit flavored and contain trace amounts of simethicone, gums, and suspending agents. Allergic reactions are rare.

Recommended Amounts for UGI Study

Newborn to 1 year	2 to 4 oz.
1 year to 3 years	4 to 6 oz.
3 years to 10 years	6 to 12 oz.
Over 10 years	12 to 16 oz.

Materials

Newborn to 3 years	Sterile 4-oz bottle with nipple. Widen nipple opening with sterile needle or scalpel.
3 years and older	Cup and/or flexible straw.

Note: Nipples and pacifiers are now available in silicone for babies allergic to latex.

Barium swallow and UGI studies are performed on children lying down. When a child is old enough to drink through a straw, the barium usually goes down easily without spilling. If a child is not able or refuses to drink through a straw, the only practical alternative is a feeding bottle because it is difficult for a patient to drink from a cup while supine. When the examination is for diagnosis of an esophageal stricture, the patient can be given a sandwich of barium paste and graham crackers.

A child with a cleft palate may need a special feeding cup. Ask the parents to bring their own. Otherwise, barium can be dripped over the back of the tongue through an 8 French feeding catheter attached to a 2-oz (60-cc) catheter tip syringe.

BARIUM SWALLOW

The use of a barium swallow depends on the age of the patient, as most esophageal abnormalities are diagnosed by the age of 1 year. Examples of reasons for conducting this examination are noisy breathing, dysphagia, vomiting, gastroesophageal reflux, aspiration, and ingestion of a corrosive chemical agent.

Possible diagnoses are a vascular ring from a double aortic arch creating esophageal and airway compression, an esophageal web, a tracheoesophageal fistula, a hiatus hernia (rare in children) and/or a foreign body.

If there is a possibility of aspiration or extravasation of contrast, such as when a child has had a recent surgical repair of a tracheoesophageal fistula, an aqueous nonionic contrast material is used instead of barium. Contrast may be injected through an 8 French feeding catheter from 10-cc syringe into the esophagus. Tracheoesophageal fistula is frequently associated with esophageal atresia, which may be diagnosed on plain radiographs.

UPPER GASTROINTESTINAL TRACT STUDY AND SMALL-BOWEL FOLLOW-THROUGH

Examples of reasons for performing the UGI study and small-bowel follow-through are projectile vomiting, bilious vomiting, abdominal pain, failure to thrive, hematemesis, and bloody stools. Possible diagnoses are pyloric stenosis, peptic ulcer, malrotation, malabsorption syndrome, Crohn disease, and cystic fibrosis.

DOUBLE-CONTRAST UPPER GASTROINTESTINAL TRACT STUDY

The double-contrast UGI study is not a common pediatric radiologic procedure. Most clinical situations do not require this examination, and it is difficult to get a child to swallow a very fizzy drink. If they do swallow it, they soon burp, and much of the gas is lost. Children normally have a fairly large amount of gas in their stomach. If additional air is necessary, for example when diagnosing a peptic ulcer, they can slurp the barium through a straw that is only half in the barium or that has a hole punctured in its side. These techniques provide enough air to give adequate double contrast.

STANDARD POSITIONING OF THE PATIENT DURING FLUOROSCOPY

1. Supine to evaluate diaphragm movement.
2. Anteroposterior and left side down, true lateral, to evaluate the upper esophagus.
3. Supine left posterior oblique, to examine the fundus of the stomach.
4. Right anterior oblique. Barium in antrum; to evaluate gastric emptying.
5. Right side down true lateral, to evaluate the duodenal loop, duodenojejunal junction, and the ligament of Treitz.
6. Prone, to examine the duodenojejunal junction in the left upper quadrant.

Radiologists tend to follow this particular sequence, because once a child turns onto the right side, the stomach starts to empty fairly quickly. It is important to identify the duodenojejunal junction before the jejunal loops fill and the area is obscured by barium. Children who become anxious or stressed when held down may develop pylorospasm, which will delay stomach emptying.

Patients referred for small-bowel follow-through will have sequential radiographs taken at 20- and 30-minute intervals until the barium reaches the ileocecal region.

ROUTINE PROJECTIONS

With today's modern equipment, permanent images can be acquired during fluoroscopy. Follow-up radiographs, if needed, would include either a supine anteroposterior or a prone posteroanterior view of the abdomen to include the stomach, centered at the lower costal margin. The radiologist may request a right anterior oblique view centered at the same level. It is helpful to ask the radiologist to point out the level of the stomach on an individual patient.

Follow-up radiographs for study of the small bowel are usually taken at 20- to 30-minute intervals (depending on transit time) until barium reaches the ileocecal valve. Transit time for infants is from 1 to 2 hours, depending on the patient's age and the condition. Strictures due to Crohn disease, for example, will slow the barium's movement. The position of the patient for sequential radiographs may alternate between supine and prone, depending on the condition of the patient and the preference of the radiologist. Fluoroscopy is repeated and spot films taken when the barium reaches the ileocecal region.

LARGE BOWEL SINGLE AND DOUBLE CONTRAST

PATIENT PREPARATION

Patient Preparation for Large Bowel Single and Double Contrast

Newborn to 2 years	No preparation necessary.
2 years to 10 years	Low-residue meal the evening before. One bisacodyl tablet or similar laxative whole, with water, before bedtime.
If no bowel movement in the morning, a stimulant enema such as a Pedi-Fleet may be given on the advice of a physician.	
10 years to adult	Same as above, except patient should take 2 bisacodyl tablets the night before. (See Appendices A and B)

Preparation of patients with acute surgical conditions and/or inflammatory bowel diseases should be done only on the advice of the referring physician. Preparation is not recommended for patients with Hirschsprung disease because cathartics clear out the impacted stool, allowing the distended portion of bowel above the narrowed segment to collapse and increasing the probability of a false-negative study. Patients who may have polyps and who are scheduled for a double-contrast enema need more stringent bowel cleansing (see Appendix B).

MATERIALS (Fig. 4–3)

1. Pediatric flexible enema tips. Balloon-type enema tips are contraindicated for pediatric patients because they may perforate the rectum or artificially distend the narrowed rectum in patients with Hirschsprung disease.[1] A variety of enema tips for pediatric patients are commercially available. Examples are pediatric Flexi-Tips made by E-Z-M (Westbury, NY) or French red Robinson catheters with metal washers placed an appropriate distance from the tip.[1] These catheters are designed to prevent insertion of the tip beyond the rectum. Nonlatex tips are recommended because of reported allergies to latex and the potential life-threatening nature of the allergic reactions, which range from mild skin irritations to anaphylactic shock.

2. Disposable enema bag with 16-oz barium sulfate, tubing, and clamp. Dilution 30% weight/volume, 25% weight/weight, 1500 mL, or according to a particular manufacturer's instructions, and mixed with warm water. The amount is variable depending on the age and condition of the child.

3. For neonates and infants: A 2-oz (60-cc) catheter tip syringe with a 10 French flexible silicone catheter. A 12 Foley catheter works well, but DO NOT INFLATE the balloon. At Children's Hospital we occasionally use an extracorporeal chest catheter with a flange as an infant enema tip. We inject the barium manually, very slowly.

4. High-density unit dose air-contrast enema kit or a regular enema bag with a double-line tip and an air insufflation device.

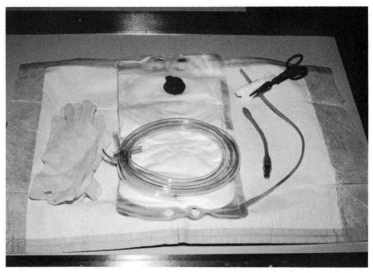

Figure 4–3
A disposable enema bag with tubing and barium; disposable gloves; a disposable flexible enema tip; and a padded, flanged catheter with a clamp for use on neonates.

5. Water-soluble lubricating jelly.
6. Hypoallergenic tape.
7. Gloves.
8. Towels and washcloths.

Run the barium through the tubing to displace air before inserting the tip into the rectum. Most children are capable of retaining barium if it is warmed and run in slowly. If not, the buttocks can be taped together to hold the tube in place. Hypoallergenic tape is best for a baby's sensitive skin and prevents welts from forming when the tape is removed. Barium is administered by gravity 3 feet above the tabletop (the recommended height). The rate of flow can be adjusted by opening the clamp only partially or by compressing the tube slightly as the barium runs in.

FLUOROSCOPY PROCEDURE

Fluoroscopy starts with the patient in the lateral position to visualize the rectum. The patient is then turned from side to side until the colon is filled and barium refluxes into the ileum. Spot films are taken during the procedure.

When a double-contrast study is performed, anteroposterior supine, posteroanterior prone, and right and left lateral decubitus radiographs are taken after air has been introduced into the bowel. Angled projections of the sigmoid region are rarely required in children. A postevacuation anteroposterior supine radiograph of the abdomen is taken to show elimination of the barium.

Generally, children do not have as much difficulty as adults—particularly the elderly—in retaining barium, except when the double-contrast study is used. Few, if any, overhead radiographs are taken until the barium or other contrast has been evacuated. The elaborate precautions taken with adults to prevent spillage onto the x-ray table is unnecessary, and cleanup in most cases is minimal.

WATER-SOLUBLE CONTRAST ENEMA

1. Diatrizoate meglumine and diatrizoate sodium solution. An enema using diatrizoate meglumine and diatrizoate sodium solution may be performed for therapeutic reduction of meconium ileus or meconium plug syndrome. In this case, the hyperosmolality of diatrizoate meglumine and diatrizoate sodium solution acts as a lavage, drawing water into the bowel and washing out the meconium. The contrast medium is diluted 50% with sterile water, warmed, put into an empty disposable enema bag, and then introduced into the colon in the same way as barium is. To prevent dehydration, the patient must be on a saline or dextrose intravenous drip before the procedure is started.

2. Isotonic contrast. Isotonic contrast, an aqueous contrast medium similar to that used for cystography, may be used instead of barium for patients with suspected perforation or chronic inflammatory bowel disease. However, the trend today is to evaluate these patients by colonoscopy rather than by a contrast enema.

3. Nonionic contrast. Nonionic contrast is preferred for neonates and infants because of its low toxicity. The contrast medium is injected very slowly through a catheter such as a 12 Foley (DO NOT INFLATE the balloon) from a 2-oz (60-cc) catheter tip syringe.

REDUCTION OF INTUSSUSCEPTION

Intussusception occurs when a portion of the large bowel telescopes into the adjacent bowel. The telescoped portion is called the intussusceptum, and the bowel surrounding it is the intussuscipiens. Children who have intussusception range in age from newborn to adolescent, but most cases occur before the age of 2 years.[1] A soft-tissue mass can usually be identified at the site of the intussusception on plain radiographs of the abdomen.[1]

Traditionally, intussusception has been reduced by barium enema under fluoroscopy (Fig. 4–4), although water-soluble contrast has also been used. Reduction of intussusception is considered successful when there has been a free flow of contrast into the terminal ileum. A postevacuation radiograph should always be taken to document a successful reduction.

Pneumatic reduction has been popular in China for a number of years and has been gaining acceptance in the United States. Because there is always a risk of perforating the gut when reducing an intussusception, air lowers the risk of fecal contamination and the added complication of barium leakage into the peritoneum.[2] Other advantages include the following: (1) It is quicker; (2) fluoroscopic time is shorter, thereby reducing patient dose; (3) the success rate is higher, and (4) intraluminal pressure is monitored.[1]

Materials

An air insufflation device such as the Shiels Intussusception Air Reduction System consists of a reusable handheld air insufflator and aneroid pressure gauge, disposable tubing, a three-way stopcock with a protective filter, vinyl discs, and an enema tip (Fig. 4–5). The stopcock allows for immediate decompression at any time during the procedure.[2]

Attached to the enema tip is a small, thin, vinyl rubber disc. The disc helps to seal the anus and prevents loss of air when it is taped to the buttocks. The radiologist

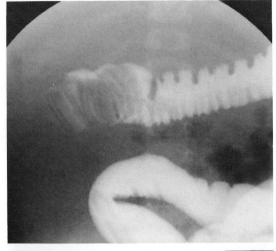

A

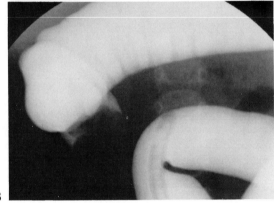

B

Figure 4–4

Reduction of intussusception by barium enema under fluoroscopy. **A**, Barium in the transverse colon at the site of obstruction. **B**, Barium has advanced to the ascending colon, gradually pushing out the telescoped bowel.

terminates the procedure if, after three attempts of 3 minutes each, with mean insufflation pressures of 120 mm Hg, the intussusception persists.[1] Successful reduction is demonstrated by a free flow of air into the small bowel and disappearance of the soft-tissue mass, the site of the intussusception[2] (Fig. 4–6).

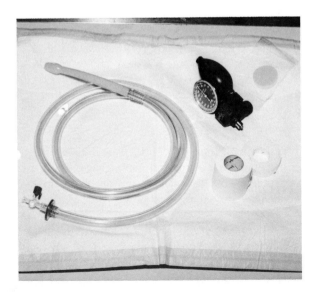

Figure 4–5

A Shiels Intussusception Air Reduction System consisting of a reusable handheld air insufflator and aneroid pressure gauge, an enema tip, vinyl discs, tape, and disposable tubing with a three-way stopcock. (The Shiels System is made by Custom Medical Products, Inc., P.O. Box 4761, Maineville, Ohio 45039.)

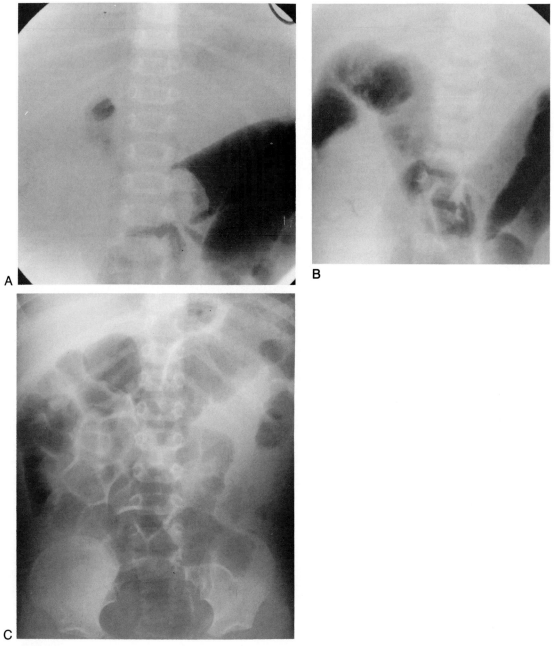

Figure 4–6
Reduction of intussusception by air enema under fluoroscopy. **A**, Air in the transverse colon, at the most common site of intussusception. **B**, Air has moved into the ascending colon, gradually pushing out the telescoped bowel. **C**, Reduction of intussusception, with air in the terminal ileum.

FLUOROSCOPY AND RADIATION DOSE

Because of their projected life span, children who have radiographic or fluoroscopic examinations early in life have a greater potential than adults for increased cumulative exposure to radiation. Fluoroscopic procedures tend to involve greater doses of radiation than do most routine radiographic procedures and, depending on the examination, a higher dose to the gonads. Preparing children for a fluoroscopic procedure and obtaining their cooperation is one way of reducing fluoroscopic time and minimizing the radiation dose.

Fluoroscopy should be intermittent rather than continuous, and the beam should be collimated to the area of interest. A visible digital counter on the television monitor, which shows elapsed seconds, is a constant reminder of fluoroscopic time to the fluoroscopist. This is preferable to relying on the signal and reset button usually located on the control panel, which is calibrated in 5-minute intervals. The shortest image intensifier to patient distance should always be used, as the greater this distance, the higher the patient dose.

The National Council on Radiation Protection and Measurements report on radiation protection in pediatric radiology[3] recommends that image intensifiers with television monitors always be used when examining children, because this equipment allows for better visualization and, in most cases, a lower dose rate. Imaging intensifiers with digital spot imaging and fluoroscopic microprocessing also reduce the radiation dose by storing images during fluoroscopy. These can be retrieved by laser imagery when the examination is completed.

The patient's fluoroscopic time should always be recorded on the requisition or the report for permanent documentation in the medical record.

REFERENCES

1. Kirks, D.R., Caron, K.H., Gastrointestinal tract, in Practical Pediatric Imaging: Diagnostic Radiology of Infants and Children, 2nd ed., pp. 708–903, D. Kirks, ed., Little, Brown & Company, Boston, 1991
2. Shiels, W.E., Bissett, G.S., and Kirks, D.R., Simple device for air reduction of intussusception, Pediatric Radiology, 20:472–474, 1990
3. National Council on Radiation Protection and Measurements, No. 68, Washington, DC, 1981

Chapter 5

The Urinary System

Normal and Abnormal Development

Excretory Urogram (IVP)
Patient Preparation
Materials
Contrast Media
Medications Readily Available for Contrast Reactions
Gonadal Shielding
Routine and Additional Projections
Scheduling

Voiding Cystourethrogram (VCUG)
Patient Preparation
Materials
Contrast Media
Recorded Information
Latex Allergy
Radionuclide Cystogram
Ultrasonography

NORMAL AND ABNORMAL DEVELOPMENT

The urinary and genital systems are closely related embryologically and anatomically. Malformation of one, as a result of abnormal embryonic development, can affect the other. These two systems develop from the embryonic intermediate mesoderm, which is also the source of blood cells, bone marrow, and the skeleton.[1]

The urinary tract consists of the kidneys, ureters, urinary bladder, and urethra. Initially in the developing embryo, the rudimentary kidneys lie close to each other in the pelvis in front of the sacrum.[1] As the abdomen and the ureters grow, the kidneys gradually "ascend" until they occupy their normal anatomic position on the posterior abdominal wall at the level of the second lumbar vertebra. Abnormalities of the kidneys and ureters occur in 3% to 4% of the population.[1] Duplication of the ureter and renal pelvis is an example of a common malformation (Fig. 5–1).

In infants and children, the urinary bladder, even when empty, is at a higher level than in adults. The urethral opening into the bladder is at the level of the upper border of the symphysis pubis and gradually sinks, assuming its adult anatomic position at puberty.[1]

Urinary tract infection (UTI) is a common problem in young children. Frequently, urinary tract infections occur in children who also have vesicoureteral reflux (backflow of urine from the bladder into the ureter and kidney) (Fig. 5–2). Reflux is usually the result of an abnormality at the junction of the ureter or ureters with the urinary bladder. Normally there is an intrinsic muscular valve, which ensures the urine flows in one direction only, from the ureter to the bladder.

Congenital shortening or absence of the submucosal portion of a ureter will allow a retrograde flow of urine from the bladder to the ureter and then into the kidney. This backflow in a child who also has a UTI can result in the transmission of bacteria from the bladder to the kidney, resulting in pyelonephritis. Recurrent kidney infections can cause renal scarring and, eventually, so much destruction of the kidney that renal function is compromised.

Treatment depends on the severity of the reflux and the age and sex of the child. Girls have more infections than boys. Minor reflux in an infant or young child may subside spontaneously. Reflux is graded I through V according to an international grading system. This facilitates comparing reflux among patients or following the progress in the same child over time[2] (Fig. 5–3). A patient with severe reflux and renal

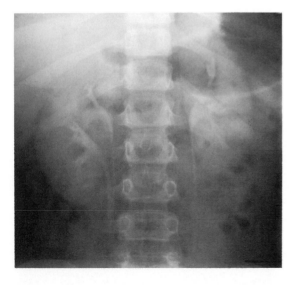

Figure 5–1

Duplication of the right ureter and the renal pelvis.

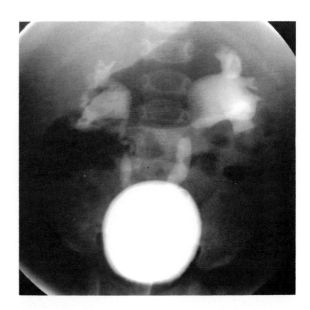

Figure 5-2
Bilateral vesicoureteral reflux in
an 18-month-old female.

scarring is a possible candidate for ureteral reimplantation, a common surgical procedure at Children's Hospital.

Renal agenesis is the congenital absence of a kidney or kidneys. The absence of
one kidney is uncommon, occurring in 1 in 1,000 infants.[1] Absence of both kidneys is
not compatible with life. An ectopic kidney is one that is in an abnormal position,
usually in the pelvis. A horseshoe-shaped kidney is one in which the lower poles of the
kidneys are fused (Fig. 5-4).

Childhood polycystic disease is inherited and is said to be due to the abnormal
development of the kidney collecting tubules.[1] The kidneys are enlarged and contain
multiple cysts, and renal function may be impaired. Polycystic disease ranges from mild
to severe and may require a renal transplant in the severe cases.

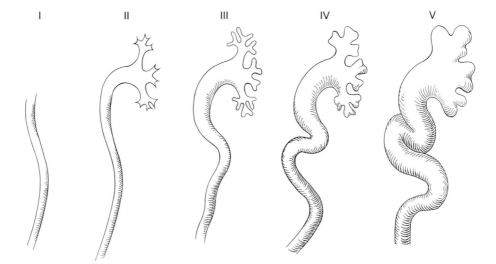

Figure 5-3
Vesicoureteral reflux is graded I through V according to severity. Grade I does not reach the
renal pelvis, whereas grade V shows gross dilatation of the ureter and the renal pelvis. (Courtesy of Robert L. Lebowitz, MD.)

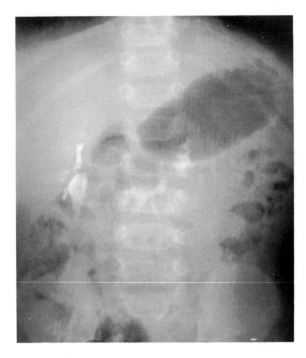

Figure 5-4
Horseshoe/crossed   ectopic   left
kidney.

Indications for examination of the urinary tract in children include abdominal masses, trauma, genital abnormalities, renal stones, and neurogenic bladder dysfunction due to a myelomeningocele. Wilms' tumor, a malignant tumor of the kidney, is the most common malignancy of childhood; 78% of cases are detected between the ages of 1 and 5 years, with a peak incidence between ages 2 and 3 years.[3] There are various imaging procedures for demonstrating anatomy and function, but the most commonly performed procedures are excretory urography, more familiarly known and referred to as intravenous pyelography (IVP); voiding cystourethrography (VCUG); radionuclide cystography; and renal ultrasonography. The choice and order of imaging depends (among other things) on the age of the child, the symptoms, and the likelihood of finding an abnormality.[4]

EXCRETORY UROGRAM (IVP)

Before beginning an examination in which intravenous contrast is used, it is important to establish (as with adults) whether the child has a history of allergies. However, studies have found fewer and less severe adverse reactions to iodinated contrast media in children. The Society for Pediatric Radiology adopted the findings of a 1974 study, which stated that because of the low adverse reaction rate, "formalized informed consent is not necessary for this relatively common and generally innocuous procedure."[5] The Department of Radiology at Children's Hospital has elected to use nonionic, low-osmolality contrast media for all patients undergoing IVP or enhanced computed tomography.

The appropriate medications and emergency procedures should always be in place when intravenous contrast is used, and a team should be ready to react swiftly. The type of reaction should be well documented for future reference, as these children frequently need follow-up studies.

When the preliminary radiograph has been taken and reviewed by a radiologist, the child should be prepared for the injection. The patient should be asked to empty the bladder before going into the injection room. The syringe should be filled, with the needle attached and out of sight. This is the time to explain the procedure to a young child. Most preschoolers become hysterical when they know they are going to receive a needle stick, so it is better not to give them much time to think about it. Older (school-age) children should be prepared beforehand. They can be given the information, and time for questions should be allowed.

Allow the mother or father, or both if they wish, to stay with the child and hold his/her hand. (I have seen an adult faint, but this is a rare occurrence and embarrasses the parent rather than hinders the procedure.) It is better not to have a parent hold a child down; this may have repercussions later. Emphasize to both the patient and parents how important it is to keep still and that this is the most difficult part of the examination.

Distractions help. The room should be painted in warm colors and have pictures on the walls. Let the child bring a favorite toy or blanket into the room. Have music playing softly in the background; a radio is always playing in these procedure rooms at Children's Hospital.

Older children may like to count, having been told the procedure will be over by the time they reach 20 or any other appropriate number. Reassure them that it is okay to cry or say "Ouch," but do not say (even to an older child), "Don't be a baby." Provide constant reassurance and keep telling them how well they are doing.

When the injection is finished, give them a Band-Aid to show off as evidence of having been through the ordeal. Give them stickers as a reward even if they screamed loudly. Stickers are readily available, safe, and inexpensive.

Because of the types of diseases and conditions they have, fewer radiographs are generally taken on children than adults. The exact number will vary, depending on the diagnosis and the radiologist. We make every attempt at Children's Hospital to take only two or three films per IVP.

Patients are encouraged to drink fluids such as water, juice, or ginger ale after the first postinjection radiograph has been taken. A nurse or attending physician should be consulted if the child is on an intravenous solution or if fluid intake is being monitored.

Children should not be expected to stay on the x-ray table while radiographs are being reviewed, unless tomography is being performed, or if the patient is too sick or handicapped to be moved easily. Young children will not remain lying down and would rather sit or be held by their mother. Older children may want to watch television while waiting for the next radiograph to be taken.

PATIENT PREPARATION

The recommended physical preparation of young children for an IVP is simple. The patient should drink plenty of clear fluids before the examination (i.e., hydration, not dehydration). The most common reaction to contrast media in children is nausea and vomiting. Solid foods should be avoided 4 hours before the examination to diminish the risk of aspiration. Fluids also should be avoided immediately before the examination.

The preparation sheet at Children's Hospital suggests that the fluids not include milk or apple juice (see Appendix B). This is not based on scientific fact but was included at the suggestion of radiographers experienced in performing an IVP in children. The radiographers had noticed that children who vomited after an injection of an iodinated contrast medium seemed to be those who had had milk or apple juice before the examination. However, if a nonionic, low-osmolality contrast medium is used, this problem is minimized, and at Children's Hospital nausea and vomiting is now rare.

Laxatives should not be given to infants or young children to clear the bowel of stool. The radiologist in charge of uroradiology at Children's Hospital has said that laxatives cause unnecessary discomfort. If there is stool in the bowel and it interferes with visualization of the urinary tract, tomograms can be performed. In earlier years, radiologists were more interested in the nephrogram to visualize the renal parenchyma, which now can be evaluated by ultrasound.

Emotional support and preparation are most important. It is always best to be truthful when telling children about the procedure. However, it is not advisable to tell toddlers that they are going to have a needle stick before going into the procedure room. Once a child is in the room, it is advisable to explain that he/she will feel a little prick or pinch on the arm or on the back of the hand, depending on the injection site.

School-age children generally handle the situation better when they are told directly that they are going to receive an injection, but it is a good idea to consult the parents beforehand, as they are more familiar with their child's emotional makeup. Keep in mind that many adults do not like needles and they may have passed this fear onto their children.

Keep needles and syringes out of sight in the room where the injection will be given. Butterfly needles should be used for tiny veins, as they are more easily kept in place and perhaps do not appear as menacing as the standard kind.

All children capable of understanding should be prepared for a visit to the hospital and the radiology department. Information, rather than lack of it, decreases anxiety. To some extent, the timing of the discussion about the visit can be left to the parent or guardian, depending on the individual child. The coordinator of the preadmission program at Children's Hospital suggests one day's notice for each year of life, but temperament rather than age seems to be the most important determinant.

Parents or guardians should have the examination explained to them in advance; for example, why it is necessary to avoid solid foods and how long they should expect to be in the department.

Appendix A contains explanatory preparation sheets originally written by college students who were once patients at Children's Hospital. As children, they had undergone many of these examinations. These simple explanation sheets were written for school-age children, and many parents find them helpful in understanding the procedure as they read them to their children.

MATERIALS

Syringes: 1, 5, 10, 20, and 50 cc. (Note: 50-cc syringes are hard to push when using viscous contrast materials and small needles.)

Butterfly needles with connecting tubing: 19, 23, 25, and 27 G. (23- and 25-G needles tend to be used the most; 27-G needles are for premature babies and very small veins; 19-G needles are large and are rarely used).

Conventional needles: 16 G and 18 G to draw up or put contrast material into an intravenous drip.

Gloves (*always* used when injecting).

Tourniquets.

Alcohol swabs.

Band-Aids.

CONTRAST MEDIA

High-osmolality contrast may be meglumine diatrizoate and sodium diatrizoate, such as Renografin, Urografin, or MD-60.

Low-osmolality, nonionic contrast may be ioversol, iopamidol, or iohexol, such as Optiray, Isovue, or Omnipaque.

CONTRAST MEDIUM DOSAGE

Weight (lb)	Dose
Up to 12	2 cc/lb
13–25	25 cc
26–50	1 cc/lb
51–100	50 cc
Over 100	½ cc/lb

Courtesy of the Radiology Department, Children's Hospital, Boston, Massachusetts.

Weight (kg)	Dose
0–5	3 ml/kg
6–15	15 ml
16–20	20 ml
21–25	25 ml
26–35	30 ml
36–45	35 ml
46–55	40 ml
56–65	45 ml
66+	50 ml (not less than 0.7 ml/kg)

Courtesy of the Radiology Department, The Hospital for Sick Children, Toronto, Ontario, Canada.

Although contrast reactions occur less frequently in children than in adults, resuscitation equipment and the appropriate medications for a minor or major reaction should be readily available. Children most often complain of feeling warm or slightly nauseous and should be reassured that these feelings will quickly go away.

MEDICATIONS READILY AVAILABLE FOR CONTRAST REACTIONS

Epinephrine, 1:1000 aqueous subcutaneous injection (1 mg/ml).
Diphenhydramine hydrochloride (Benadryl), for injection (50 mg/ml) and by mouth (elixir, 1 tsp = 12.5 mg).

GONADAL SHIELDING

Males, in nearly all instances, can be shielded for all radiographs because the testes lie outside the abdominal cavity.

Females should be shielded for the 3-minute kidney radiograph and for tomograms of the kidneys. If the ovaries are shielded correctly, the lower ureters and bladder are obscured. Gonadal shielding, or lack of it, should be explained carefully to the parents. Frequently, parents are concerned about the cumulative effects of radiation to their children's gonads from these examinations.

ROUTINE AND ADDITIONAL PROJECTIONS

> **Routine Projections:**
>
> 1. Scout or preliminary radiograph to include kidneys, ureters, and bladder (Fig. 5–5A).
> 2. Three minutes after injection, kidneys only (Fig. 5–5B).
> 3. Fifteen minutes after injection, anteroposterior (supine) or posteroanterior (prone) of kidneys, ureters, and bladder (Fig. 5–5C).
>
> Separate radiographs of the bladder are rarely needed in children.

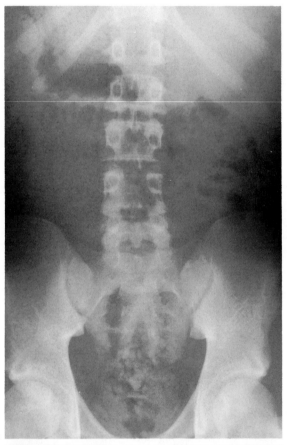

A

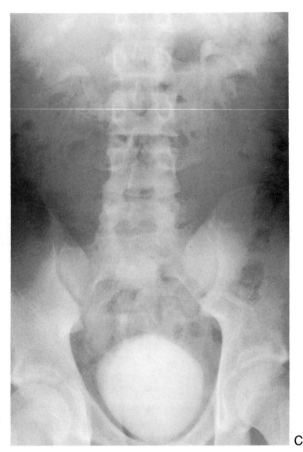

C

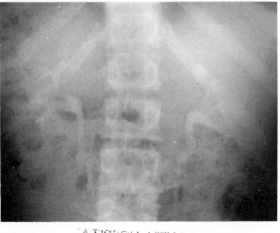

B

Figure 5–5

Normal excretory urogram in a 16-year-old male. **A**, Scout or preliminary film. **B**, 3-minute film of kidneys only. **C**, 15-minute film of kidneys, ureters, and bladder.

Tomography may be necessary at the time of the scout radiograph if the purpose is to look for an opaque stone, or whenever a clearer image devoid of stool is needed.

Patients undergoing radiography for the first time at Children's Hospital usually have three radiographs taken, but a patient who is being followed, for example, for postreimplantation of ureters, may need only a preliminary and a 15-minute postinjection radiograph of the kidneys, ureters, and bladder.

Some of the literature suggests giving the patient a carbonated drink after injection. This fills the stomach with gas, which pushes down on the bowel, creating a radiolucent window through which the opacified kidneys are visualized. We do not perform this procedure at Children's Hospital. The gas causes discomfort and may pass into the bowel, compounding the problem. Tomography gives as clear an image of the kidneys as the gas-filled stomach.

Upon completion of the examination, parents should be told to give their child plenty of fluids.

Technical Considerations: A 400-speed screen/film system is recommended for the best resolution at the lowest radiation dose.

SCHEDULING

Patients may be scheduled for both a VCUG and an IVP. In most instances, the IVP follows the VCUG. If kidney size and morphology rather than function is being evaluated, renal ultrasonography is performed more often than IVP and may precede or follow a VCUG, helping to reduce radiation dose. Ultrasonography is particularly useful for patients being followed for reflux. Postoperatively and for screening purposes, a radionuclide cystogram may replace the VCUG.

VOIDING CYSTOURETHROGRAM (VCUG)

The VCUG involves filling the urinary bladder with contrast material by gravity through a catheter until the patient feels the need to void. The child then voids while on the table. Fluoroscopy should be brief and intermittent to keep the radiation dose to a minimum. The VCUG should be explained beforehand to both the parent and child in simple language. Explanation sheets for both boys and girls are contained in Appendix A.

PATIENT PREPARATION

Children over age 3 may be less apprehensive if they are taken into the room beforehand and shown the equipment and how it works. They should be shown how the image intensifier is brought over them but does not get close enough to touch, squash, or injure them. They may wish to watch the television screen. Although the technical term *void* is used here, you should be prepared to use a word the child understands—preferably one that is used at home. "Pee" and "tinkle" are common, but there are many others as well. Ask the parent what term is common to their family so that the child understands what you are asking them to do.

This procedure can be as difficult and embarrassing for a young child as it is for an adult. The child should have as much privacy as possible, with few observers during the examination. It frequently takes time to initiate voiding, and it is particularly difficult for very young children who have recently been toilet trained. Asking them to void onto a table lying down after having been trained to sit or stand can be difficult to justify or explain.

The procedure should not be uncomfortable for the patient. Potential discomfort in boys should be prevented by using 2% lidocaine (Xylocaine) jelly to locally anesthetize the urethra prior to the insertion of the catheter.

This procedure requires no special preparation other than asking the patient to empty his/her bladder before starting the examination. A parent should accompany an infant or young child into the procedure room. Older children, particularly teenagers, may prefer to be on their own. The child is asked to lie supine on the fluoroscopy table; girls assume a frog-leg position.

The perineum is then cleansed with an antiseptic antimicrobial skin cleanser (such as Hibiclens or Betadine), which is then washed away with sterile saline. Both solutions

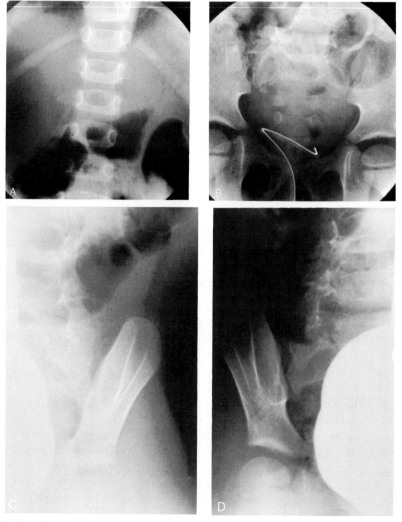

Figure 5-6

Normal voiding cystourethrogram of a 3-year-old female. **A**, Scout or preliminary film of the kidney area. **B**, Scout film of the urinary bladder. **C** and **D**, Right and left oblique views of the vesicoureteral region.

should be warmed. If the area around the meatus is irritated or erythematous, 2% lidocaine jelly can be applied before cleansing to prevent stinging.[4]

Most children can be catheterized with an 8 French feeding tube lubricated with 2% lidocaine jelly, although a 5 French may be needed for premature babies. A retaining catheter (such as a Foley) should not be used for this procedure in children. Residual urine collected through the catheter should be sent to the laboratory for a culture.

The bladder is filled slowly by gravity with a dilute contrast material, about 17% weight/volume, to minimize irritation of the bladder wall and possible chemical cystitis. When bladder capacity is approached, gravity filling will slow and then stop automatically.[2] Bladder capacity is determined by the patient's age. In infants under 1 year, the weight in kilograms times 7 equals the capacity in milliliters. In children over 1 year, the age in years plus 2, times 30, has been predicted to be the capacity in milliliters.[3] Some manufacturers supply bottles of contrast in two sizes: 250 cc and 500 cc.

When it has been determined that the bladder is full, the child is asked to void and should be voiding before the catheter is removed. This part of the procedure can take time, although running faucets and dripping warm water onto the perineum will usually start the process.

Images recorded during fluoroscopy include the following:

1. Scout radiograph of the kidneys and bladder before contrast is instilled (Fig. 5–6A and B).
2. Right and left oblique views of the bladder when full to show the vesicoureteral regions (Fig. 5–6C and D).
3. Urethra while voiding (Fig. 5–6E).
4. Postvoid radiograph of the bladder and kidneys (Fig. 5–6F).

A radiograph is sometimes taken during early filling of the bladder to show or rule out a ureterocele. More radiographs may be taken when an abnormality is discovered.

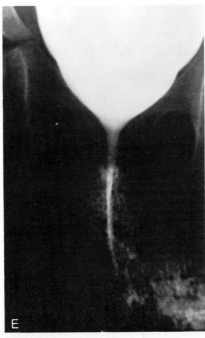
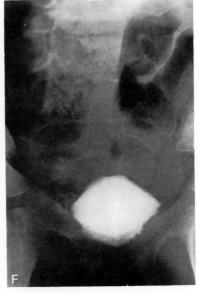

Figure 5–6 *Continued*
E, The urethra during voiding. *F,* The urinary bladder after voiding.

When the procedure is completed, the child should be told to drink plenty of water or a favorite soda or juice for the remainder of the day to minimize postprocedural dysuria (difficult or painful urination). The parent and child should be advised that a burning sensation may occur when urinating and the urine may be pink. This is not unusual, and drinking plenty of fluids will help resolve these problems quickly.

MATERIALS

Sterile tray with three small bowls, cotton balls, and a clamp.
Sterile gauze.
Sterile container for collecting a urine specimen from the catheter.
8 French feeding tube.
Sterile water, warmed.
2% lidocaine jelly.
Antiseptic skin cleanser, warmed.
Gloves.
Towels.
Urine receptacle.

For boys over age 3, the tray should include a 10-cc syringe and a fistula tip.

CONTRAST MEDIA

Contrast such as iothalamate meglumine, 17.2% for cystography.

CONTRAST MEDIUM DOSAGE	
Age (yr)	Dose (cc)
Under 2	250
Over 2	500

RECORDED INFORMATION

The following information should be recorded:

Quantity of residual urine, which should be sent to the laboratory for a culture.
Predicted bladder capacity.
Volume and type of contrast used.
Fluoroscopy time.

LATEX ALLERGY

Recent studies[6] have shown that patients who are constantly exposed to rubber catheters and rubber gloves may develop allergies to latex. For example, patients with neurogenic bladder dysfunction, who have numerous operations and must frequently catheterize themselves, become sensitized by the constant touching. The allergic response ranges in severity from hives and sneezing to difficulty in breathing and anaphylactic shock. It is now considered advisable to use silicone or Silastic catheters

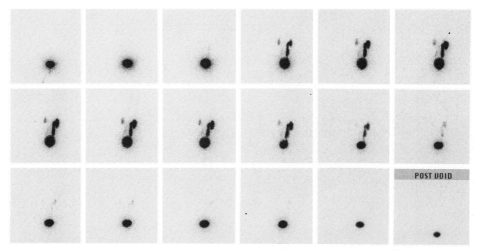

POST VOID

Figure 5–7

Radionuclide cystogram showing the bladder filling with bilateral reflux (greater on the right than on the left), gradually emptying, and after voiding. (In scintigraphy the camera is beneath the patient, and the urinary tract is viewed from the back.)

and nonlatex gloves, particularly with patients whose condition predisposes them to become sensitized to rubber.

RADIONUCLIDE CYSTOGRAM

Radionuclide cystograms show and confirm reflux but do not demonstrate the anatomic detail seen on VCUGs (Fig. 5–7). The radiation dose is much lower than for a VCUG. A radionuclide cystogram may be performed as a follow-up after surgery (for example, after reimplantation of ureters), for family screening, and for follow-up of reflux being managed nonoperatively.[2]

Preparation for a radionuclide cystogram is similar to that for a fluoroscopic VCUG. The child first empties the bladder, then lies on a table over a gamma camera, and is prepared and catheterized. Residual urine is collected, measured, and sent to the laboratory for a culture. One millicurie of ^{99m}Tc pertechnetate is then instilled, followed by sterile water until the bladder is full and the child voids. Radioisotope in the ureters and kidneys indicates reflux.

ULTRASONOGRAPHY

IVP, VCUG, and radionuclide cystogram studies are invasive procedures and involve ionizing radiation. Ultrasonography of the kidneys and urinary bladder is noninvasive, requires no contrast, is painless, and is becoming increasingly important in pediatric imaging. Ultrasonography is performed to show kidney size and position, parenchymal thickness, echotexture, and dilatation of the pelvicalyceal system and ureter[3] (Fig. 5–8).

Allow children to feel the transducer and touch the gel before ultrasonography begins, so they know what it will feel like on their bellies. It is also a good idea to do the ultrasonogram before an invasive procedure such as a cystogram is performed.

The bladder is scanned first, while it is full, to look for signs of cystitis such as thickening of the bladder wall or bladder stones, particularly in infants, who sometimes

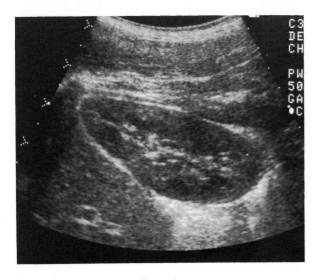

Figure 5-8
Normal prone longitudinal ultrasound scan of the right kidney.

void when the transducer is pressed on their lower abdomens. Longitudinal and transverse scans of both kidneys are done to measure kidney size and to see the parenchyma. Kidney measurements are from upper to lower poles and should be within the prescribed limits for patient size and age (Fig. 5-9).

The imaging tests described in this chapter are performed for reasons other than to detect a urinary tract infection, but the approach to the child and the procedure is much the same. The information comes mainly from the team of radiographers who perform the examinations at Children's Hospital. This team works closely with the staff uroradiologist. The radiographers are trained to inject IVPs on children of all age groups and to catheterize, fluoroscope, and scan early teenage and adolescent females for VCUGs and radionuclide cystograms. This approach has been used successfully for over 20 years at Children's Hospital and meets the standards of the Joint Commission on the Accreditation of Healthcare Organizations.

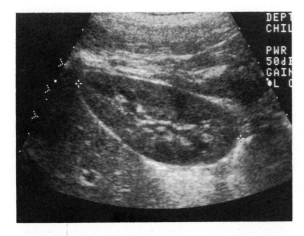

Figure 5-9
Normal prone longitudinal ultrasound scan of the right kidney. *Asterisks* on the upper and lower poles are for measuring kidney size.

REFERENCES

1. Moore, K.L., The Developing Human, W.B. Saunders Company, Philadelphia, 1988
2. Lebowitz, R.L., The detection and characterization of vesicoureteral reflux in the child, American Journal of Radiology, 148(November):1640–1642, 1992
3. Bissett, G.S., III, Strife, J.L., Kirks, D.R., Genitourinary tract, in Practical Pediatric Imaging: Diagnostic Radiology of Infants and Children, 2nd ed., pp. 904–1056, D. Kirks, ed., Little, Brown & Company, Boston, 1991
4. Lebowitz, R.L., Infection of the urinary tract in children: The role of radiology, Refresher Course on Pediatric Uroradiology, Radiological Society of North America, Oak Brook, IL, 1988
5. Gooding, C.A., Berdon, W.E., Brodeur, A.E., et al, Adverse reactions to intravenous pyelography in children, American Journal of Radiology, 123:802–804, 1975
6. Shaer, C., Slater, J.E., Latex Allergy in Children, Current Opinion in Pediatrics, 5:700–704, 1993

Chapter 6

The Appendicular Skeleton

DEVELOPMENT OF THE LONG BONES

The growing tubular bones are made up of four parts: the diaphysis or shaft, the epiphysis, the physis, and the metaphysis. These segments are not always well defined radiographically, but it is important to be aware of them and the changes that take place in growing bone (Fig. 6–1).

The long and short bones are preformed from cartilage. The primary site of ossification develops in the center of the bone, which then becomes the diaphysis. The diaphysis increases in length through the growing ends and in width through the periosteum.

Within the epiphyseal cartilage, secondary ossification centers develop at one end or both ends. The appearance and ossification of these secondary centers follow a definite pattern as the centers ossify at different but predictable times from birth to adolescence. Generally, the earlier the appearance of an epiphysis, the later it fuses with the shaft, forming the adult bone.

The physis, or growth plate, is composed of the cartilage lying between the secondary center and the metaphysis and is seen as a dark line on a radiograph. Depending on the stage of growth, this line will be irregular and may look like a fracture to those unfamiliar with pediatric radiography. The metaphysis is the area where the diaphysis gradually expands into a trumpet-like configuration as it approaches the growth plate. The dense line adjacent to the radiolucent growth plate is believed to correspond to the zone of provisional calcification, where the physeal cartilage ossifies.

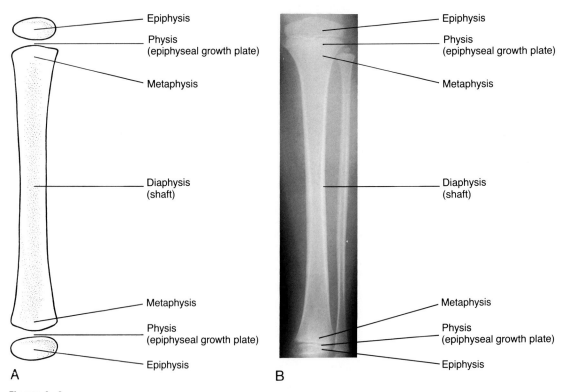

Figure 6–1

A, Diagram showing the diaphysis, epiphyses, physes, and metaphyses in the growing long bone. The diaphysis is the primary ossification center, and the epiphyses are the secondary ossification centers. **B**, Radiograph of the tibia and fibula showing the diaphysis, epiphyses, physes, and metaphyses in a 6-year-old child.

Some illnesses affect bone growth, and the slowing of growth is demonstrated on a radiograph by bands of increased density at the ends of bones. The width of the band and its distance from the end of the bone indicate the duration and the severity of a disease, similar to drought rings in the trunk of a tree.

The round bones (the carpal and tarsal bones) are rarely ossified at birth, but the calcaneus and talus are usually seen in the newborn. Fetal maturity may be indicated by the ossification of the epiphyses at the distal end of the femur and proximal tibia.

PATHOLOGY AND RADIOGRAPHIC TECHNIQUE

The bones of infants and children are not as dense as those of adults, and there is less radiographic contrast between bone and soft tissue. Small linear fractures are not always visible radiographically, and good soft-tissue detail is very important in determining the site of an injury. The displacement of a fat pad or the presence of fluid in the tissues may be the only radiographic sign of injury. These subtle changes may not seem as important as an obvious fracture, but injury to the physis can result in the retardation or cessation of growth, with subsequent shortening of bone.

About one third of skeletal injuries in children are to the growth plate, and the most common sites of growth plate fractures are the wrist and ankle.[1] In 1963, Salter and Harris described the classic five types of growth-plate fractures. A Type I fracture is a separation of the epiphysis from the growth plate; Type II fracture, the most common, occurs when the fracture extends into the metaphyseal bone on one side (Fig. 6–2); Type III fracture extends from the growth plate into the epiphysis; Type IV fracture includes both the epiphysis and metaphysis, and Type V fracture is a crush injury of the growth plate[2] (Fig. 6–3).

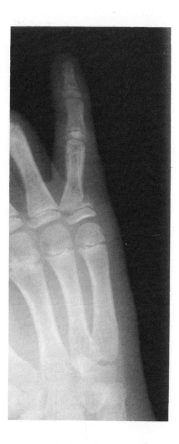

Figure 6–2
Type II fracture of the proximal phalanx of the right little finger.

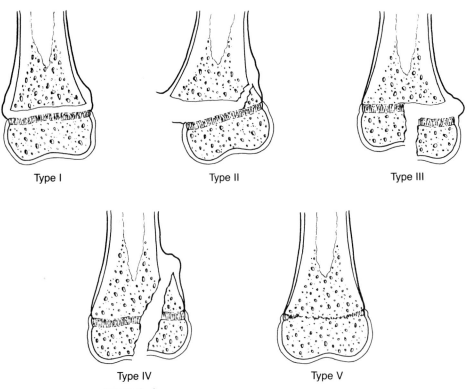

Type I   Type II   Type III

Type IV   Type V

Figure 6-3
Salter-Harris classification of growth plate fractures.

Fractures in children, as in adults, may be simple, comminuted, or open. A greenstick fracture, so called because it resembles a bent sapling, is an incomplete fracture, with bending of one side or both sides of the cortex. Greenstick fractures are most common in the radius and ulna. A buckle fracture of the distal radial metaphysis occurs frequently in children when they fall on an outstretched hand.

A very young child, when asked "Where does it hurt?," will invariably point to the whole limb. This makes it difficult to make an accurate clinical diagnosis. In earlier years, when there was less concern regarding radiation dose to the patient, the recommendation was to take radiographs of both limbs for comparison. However, radiographs showing good soft-tissue detail will, in most cases, obviate the need for comparison radiographs of the opposing limb, and radiographing both sides for comparison should never be done routinely.

Congenital deformities, osteomyelitis, arthritis, malignancies, bone cysts, deficiencies caused by malnutrition and intrauterine diseases, and changes due to endocrine malfunction are all common in children and, like trauma, may result in deformity.

Technical Considerations: For most examinations of the extremities, and when a grid is not used, a good-detail film/screen combination such as Kodak Fine with TML film is recommended. A low-contrast screen/film combination with some degree of latitude is recommended, as it assists radiographically in demonstrating the intermediate grays of the soft tissues as well as bone detail. On older patients, and when it is necessary to use a grid, a 400 rare-earth screen/film combination can be used. Whenever possible, a small focal spot and the shortest possible exposure times should be used to ensure good visibility of bone trabeculae with minimal geometric unsharpness and without motion.

RADIOGRAPHIC EXAMINATIONS

Radiographic projections and positioning of the extremities are similar for children and adults, although the clinical reasons for the examination may differ. In children, fractures are more common than sprains.[3] To demonstrate minor fractures, it is always advisable to take anteroposterior, oblique, and lateral views. The radiographer should be gentle; the fracture may not be obvious, but it still hurts, and the cooperation of the patient is desirable. Obvious fractures should always be immobilized before the patient comes to the radiology department. The following is a selection of the more common radiographic examinations requested for children.

HAND AND WRIST, AND LEFT LOWER LIMB TO ASSESS BONE AGE

A bone-age examination is performed to assess the skeletal versus the chronological age of a child from infancy through adolescence. Bones develop in an orderly pattern, and developmental delay in growth can occur because of illness, endocrine or metabolic dysfunction, and some types of medication and therapy.

The hand and wrist examination is usually the examination of choice because changes are readily visible and easily evaluated. The left hand and wrist is the standard. The International Agreement for the Unification of Anthropometric Measurements of Physical Anthropologists in 1906 and 1912 specified that measurements be made of the left side of the body, including the left extremities, rather than the right side.[4]

The examination is simple but must include all the phalanges, metacarpals, and carpals and the distal ends of the radius and ulna. Radiologists evaluating skeletal age will use a textbook such as Greulich and Pyle's, which illustrates radiographically the hand and wrist of males and females from birth to 18 years of age (Fig. 6–4).[4]

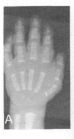
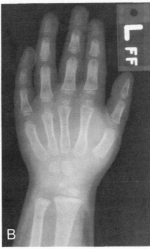
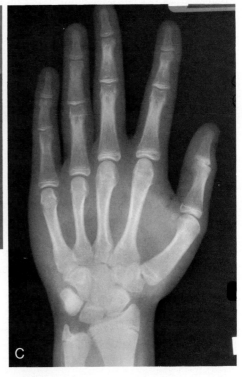

Figure 6–4
A, Hand of 1-day-old male showing capitate and hamate. **B**, Hand of 2½-year-old male whose bone age is 3³⁄₁₂ years. **C**, Hand of 14-year-old male with almost complete epiphyseal fusion.

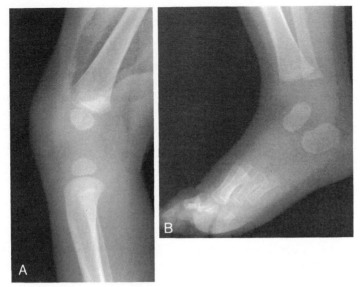

Figure 6–5
Epiphyses of the distal femur and proximal tibia (**A**) and calcaneus and talus (**B**) are present, showing appropriate skeletal development for a full-term infant.

Routine Projection: Posteroanterior, left hand and wrist.

The carpal bones are not visible in newborns or in children under 2 years of age, and relatively little change occurs in the ossification centers of the hands and wrists.[5] When assessing skeletal maturation in this age group, it is more helpful to take a lateral radiograph of the left lower limb.[5] At Children's Hospital, we routinely take a lateral radiograph of the knee, ankle, and foot in children under the age of 1 year. This will show the epiphysis of the distal femur, the proximal tibia, and the tarsal bones. Usually the calcaneus and talus are visible when the neonate is full term (Fig. 6–5).

Routine Projection: Lateral lower limb, including the knee, ankle, and foot.

WRIST

Buckle fractures of the distal radius are seen most often in preschoolers, whereas older children are more likely to sustain Salter-Harris fractures through the growth plate, as described earlier in this chapter.[6] A fracture through the growth plate with displacement will be visible on the anteroposterior and lateral projections. A buckle fracture is not always well seen and frequently requires an oblique as well as a lateral projection (Fig. 6–6).

Routine Projections: Anteroposterior or anteroposterior, oblique and lateral.

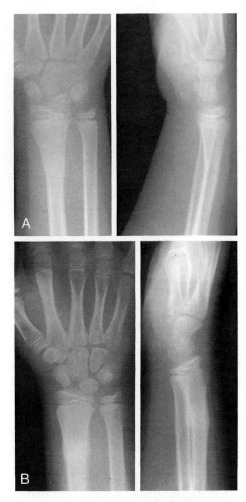

Figure 6–6
A, Anteroposterior and lateral views of the wrist, showing buckle fracture of the distal radius. **B**, Anteroposterior and lateral views of the same wrist in the healing phase. The extent of the fracture is more evident.

ELBOW

The elbow joint is a common site of injury in children, and radiologists use the "fat pad sign" in making a diagnosis. In the normal joint, the posterior fat pad lies close to the posterior surface of the distal humerus and is not normally visible on the lateral projection. A fat pad elevated because of joint effusion may be the only radiographic indication of a hairline fracture in a child or adolescent. To demonstrate this anatomic variance, it is important to be able to visualize the soft tissues and to ensure that the elbow is in a true lateral position, with the joint flexed at 90 degrees (Fig. 6–7).

A toddler may incur an injury to the elbow when an arm is jerked, dislocating the radial head, as an adult in a hurry pulls her along. Typically, the child arrives at the emergency room holding the arm slightly flexed and pronated. Often this injury is reduced by the radiographer when the elbow is supinated for the anteroposterior projection, so the radiographs look normal.

A more severe injury is the supracondylar fracture, which is the most common elbow fracture in children, accounting for approximately 60% of all pediatric elbow fractures.[7] Most are caused by falling on an outstretched hand with the elbow hyperextended. This type of fracture is seen frequently in children between the ages of 3 and 10 years.[7]

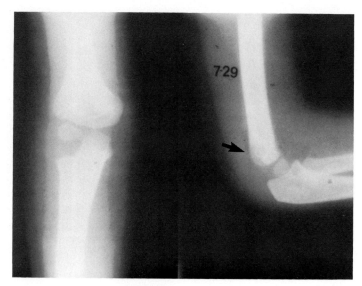

Figure 6-7
Anteroposterior and lateral views of the elbow joint. The lateral view shows the elevation of the posterior distal humerus fat pad (*arrow*) resulting from joint effusion.

The level or grade of the fracture varies from a fracture with no displacement to one involving extensive displacement of the distal humerus from the shaft (Fig. 6-8). The injury can cause serious vascular and joint complications and must be radiographed carefully and be followed by prompt orthopedic treatment. A displaced supracondylar fracture should be positioned only by an orthopedic surgeon if manipulation is necessary to obtain the right position and projection.

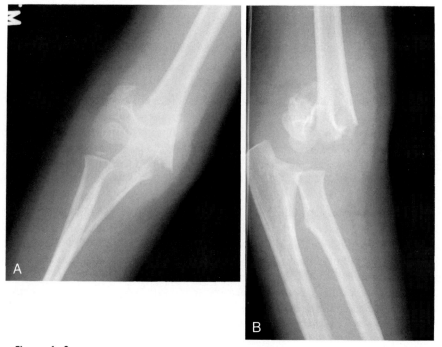

Figure 6-8
A and *B*, Supracondylar fracture with posterior displacement of the distal humerus.

> **Routine Projections:** Lateral, anteroposterior and/or axial, depending on the severity of the injury.

HUMERUS

Before adolescence, injuries to the proximal humerus are usually through or close to the growth plate between the head and the shaft. Dislocations are rare until after the epiphysis has closed in the late teens. Injuries are usually due to hyperextension of the shoulder during a fall. The head of the humerus will stay intact, while the shaft is displaced medially and posteriorly[6] (Fig. 6–9).

> **Routine Projections:** Anteroposterior and transthoracic lateral to show the shoulder joint and the upper third of the humerus.

CLAVICLE

The clavicle is a common site of fractures in children under age 10; the fracture is usually through the middle third of the shaft.[1] Whether greenstick, buckle, or complete with displacement, fractures heal and remodel quickly. In smaller children, the clavicle is generally well seen on an anteroposterior projection. The child accepts this position easily, and the radiograph can be taken either supine or erect, depending on the age and the condition of the patient (Fig. 6–10).

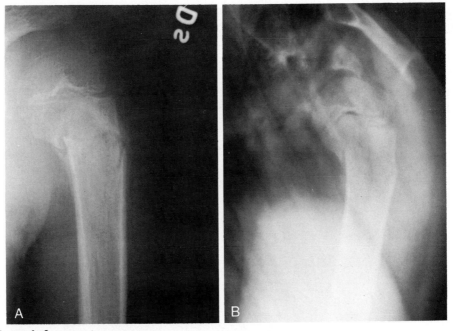

Figure 6–9

A, Anteroposterior and **B,** transthoracic lateral views showing fracture through the metaphysis of the proximal humerus close to the growth plate.

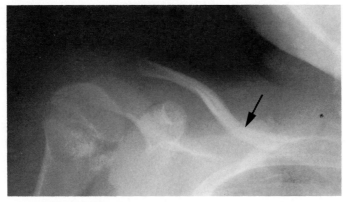

Figure 6–10
Buckle fracture (*arrow*) of the mid-third of the clavicle.

Routine Projections: Anteroposterior and/or posteroanterior. An axial view may be necessary for older children.

FOOT

Clubfoot (talipes equinovarus) is one of the most common congenital deformities in infants and occurs in 1 of every 1,000 births.[8] It is more common in boys than in girls, and in half of all children with clubfoot the condition is bilateral. In talipes equinovarus, the heel is inverted, the forefoot and midfoot are inverted and adducted, and the foot is plantar flexed, with the toes lower than the heel.[8]

To evaluate this condition and to show alignment of the calcaneus and talus and their relationship to the forefoot, weight-bearing views should be taken if the child is old enough to stand. If not, lateral radiographs should be taken with the feet in stressed dorsiflexion (Fig. 6–11). This can be accomplished by pressing a strip of plexiglass firmly against the plantar aspect of the foot (Fig. 6–12).

One method of treatment is to correct and immobilize the feet in a cast. Orthopedic surgeons do not always understand how difficult it is to produce good diagnostic radiographs of an infant's feet in a heavy cast. The problem is that the thickness of the

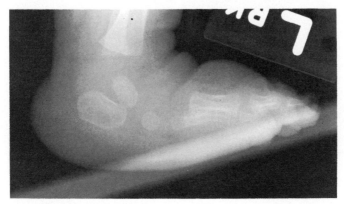

Figure 6–11
Lateral projection of a clubfoot in stressed dorsiflexion.

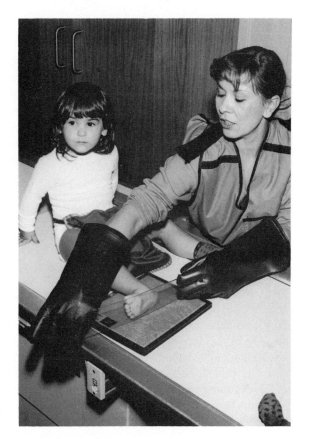

Figure 6–12
Dorsiflexion of the foot using a
plexiglass strip.

cast is often greater than the density of the bones, particularly when the bones have
been immobilized for a few months. The kilovoltage should be low—not more than 60
kvp—to avoid overpenetration, but even so, these radiographs are often
unsatisfactory.

> **Routine Projections:** Anteroposterior and lateral of both feet with stressed
> dorsiflexion, before treatment. The feet should be positioned as similarly as
> possible for comparison, and the talus and calcaneus should be visible on both
> the anteroposterior and lateral views.

BIG TOE

Stubbing injuries of the big toe in young children may result in an epiphyseal plate
fracture of the distal phalanx. Because of the proximity of the growth plate to the skin
above it, the fracture may extend to the cuticle and the root of the nail, leading to
infection and possible osteomyelitis.[9]

> **Routine Projections:** Anteroposterior oblique, and lateral.

ANKLE

In children, the ligaments of the ankle joint are stronger than bone and especially stronger than the physis.[3] Therefore, fractures are more common than sprains and frequently involve the physes of the distal tibia and fibula.[3] Fractures are classified by the Salter-Harris method described earlier in this chapter. As with the elbow joint, anteroposterior, lateral, and oblique radiographs are always required to ensure that Type I fractures of the lower end of the fibula are not missed.[1] The more severe the injury, the greater the likelihood of joint deformity (Fig. 6–13).

▼ | **Routine Projections:** Anteroposterior, lateral, and medial oblique.

TIBIA AND FIBULA

"Toddler's fracture" is a spiral fracture of the tibia that occurs in infants who are beginning to stand, walk, or run. The fracture is not always well seen radiographically until after the formation of the periosteal callus. The initial radiographs may show only swelling of the deep soft tissues—yet another example of the need for radiographs to have a long gray scale.

The clinical history may be vague and the trauma nonspecific, except that the child will refuse to bear weight on the affected leg. The medial oblique view is said to show the fewest false-negatives (Fig. 6–14).

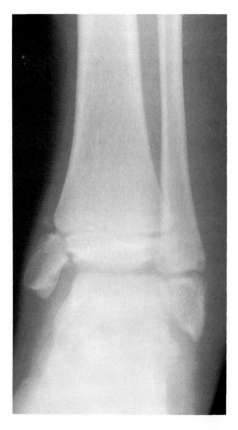

Figure 6–13

Type IV fracture of the left tibial epiphysis and epiphyseal plate.

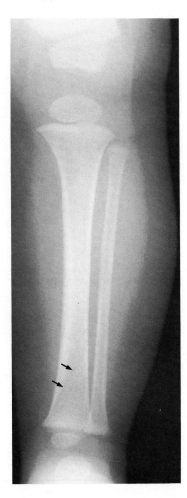

Figure 6–14
Anteroposterior view of a spiral fracture *(arrows)*
("toddler's fracture") of the distal third of the tibia.

> **Routine Projections:** Anteroposterior, lateral, and medial oblique.

KNEE

The ligaments of the knee joint are much stronger than the physis in growing bone. One of the more common injuries is an avulsion fracture of the tibial spine (Fig. 6–15). If a bony fragment becomes detached, it will become a loose body within the joint space.

> **Routine Projections:** Anteroposterior, lateral, both obliques, and axial to show the intercondylar fossa and patella. The lateral projection should be taken with a horizontal beam to detect a possible fat-fluid level seen in patients with occult fractures.

TIBIAL TUBERCLE

Patellar fractures are not common in children, but avulsion fractures of the tibial tubercle (at the insertion of the patellar tendon) occur in the early teens, when the

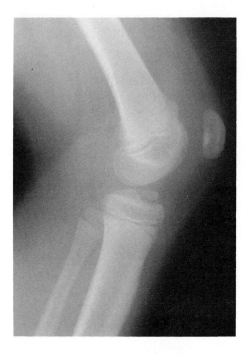

Figure 6–15
Lateral view of the left knee, showing an avulsion fracture of the tibial spine. Effusion is present in the suprapatellar pouch.

tubercle is most prominent (Fig. 6–16), before it unites with the shaft.[3] Chronic avulsion fractures occurring between ages 12 and 13 constitute Osgood-Schlatter disease. Both acute and chronic fractures are best demonstrated on the lateral radiograph of the knee.[3]

Routine Projections: Anteroposterior and lateral.

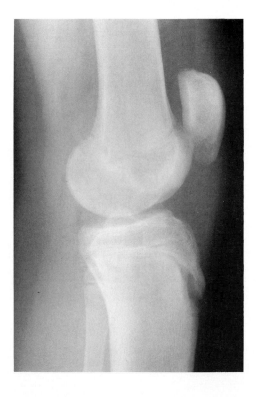

Figure 6–16
Lateral view of an avulsion fracture of the tibial tubercle.

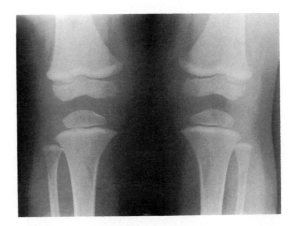

Figure 6–17
Bands of increased density at the distal ends of both femora and the proximal tibiae and fibulae, indicating lead toxicity.

KNEES FOR LEAD TOXICITY

Lead toxicity causes abnormal osteoclastic function, which results in dense bands in the metaphyses of growing bones. The width and length of the bands will depend on the amount of lead and the length of time the lead has been ingested.

An anteroposterior projection of both knees is commonly requested to evaluate a child for lead poisoning. Because there is normally some increased density at the growth plate in the femur and tibia, evaluating the proximal fibula is the best way to avoid a false-positive diagnosis. (Fig. 6–17). To determine whether a child has ingested lead (usually from lead paint chips), it may be necessary to take a plain anteroposterior supine radiograph of the abdomen. If the child has ingested lead paint, the chips will be visible in the gut.

Routine Projections: Anteroposterior of both knees and supine anteroposterior of the abdomen after recent lead ingestion.

LOWER LIMBS FOR LEG-LENGTH DISCREPANCY

A discrepancy in the length of one of the lower limbs can be corrected by either a leg-shortening or a leg-lengthening procedure. Epiphysiodesis retards the growth of the longer limb, while leg lengthening is done using a bone distraction procedure. If the disparity is small, a shoe lift will take care of the problem, but if it is severe and surgery is contemplated, accurate scanograms of the lower limbs are required.

Scanogram

There are several ways of performing scanograms; at Children's Hospital we prefer to radiograph the hips, knees, and ankles on one film using three separate exposures. With this method, two radiopaque rules are taped to the table (Fig. 6–18); no other special equipment is needed. In preparing for the procedure, it is important to note the following:

1. After being positioned on the table, the patient must not move until the three exposures are taken and the examination is completed.

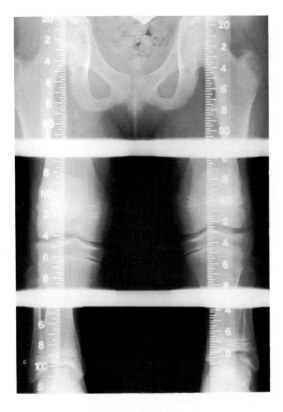

Figure 6–18

Scanogram performed with two radiopaque rules, one under each limb. Three separate exposures of the hips, knees, and ankles were taken on the same film.

2. The cassette must be marked to ensure that each collimated area does not overlap the next. Lead strips help prevent overlap fogging.

3. Centering must be directly over the joint spaces of both limbs. If the discrepancy is greater than 2.5 cm, follow the same positioning procedure, and radiograph each limb separately (Fig. 6–19).

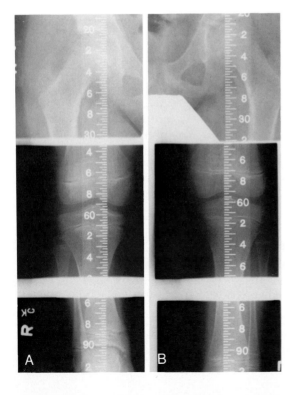

Figure 6–19

A and *B*, Scanogram performed with the limbs radiographed separately because leg-length discrepancy was greater than 2.5 cm.

4. Have technical factors ready to set for each exposure before starting the examination.

▼ **PROCEDURE**

1. Tape the scanogram rules to the table, each aligned to a limb (see Fig. 6-18).

2. Position the patient supine on the midline of the table.

3. Ensure that the hips, knees, and ankles are over the rules.

4. Place a cassette (14 by 17 in.) lengthwise in the Bucky tray.

5. Center the hip joints to the upper third of the cassette; make the exposure.

6. Slide the table up until the patient's knee joints are centered at the middle third of the cassette; reduce collimation and technique; make the exposure.

7. Slide the table up until the ankle joints are centered at the lower third of the cassette; reduce the collimation and technique; make the exposure.

The procedure is simple, and most problems arise from not having the rules and legs properly aligned. Inaccuracies also occur if both limbs are radiographed together and the patient has a leg-length discrepancy greater than 2.5 cm.

Some facilities use only one rule taped to the center of the table and follow the same radiographic procedure. One advantage of using two rules is that gonadal shielding can be used. When only one rule is used, down the center of the table, lead shielding frequently obscures the scale at the level of the hip joints.

LONG BONES AND THE BATTERED-CHILD SYNDROME

As stated in Chapter 1, children are often abused, beaten, and neglected. In 1946, John Caffey observed that fractures of the long bones were a common complication of infantile subdural hematoma. The fractures seemed to have a traumatic origin, but the traumatic episodes and the causal mechanism remained obscure.[10] In 1962, C. Henry Kempe and his associates published an article in the *Journal of the American Medical Association* entitled *The Battered Child Syndrome*. In this paper, "Kempe and his associates criticized the medical profession for its unwillingness to diagnose child abuse, which stemmed from physicians' emotional ties with the parents, denial of the facts, ignorance of their legal and moral responsibilities, and fear of being embroiled in a controversy."[11]

Pediatricians and pediatric radiologists have long been aware of unexplainable fractures in children. Parents usually denied occurrence of any specific accident or injury, and these injuries were attributed to a child's "soft" bones or propensity for falling down. Once Kempe described the "battered-child syndrome" and the pattern of trauma observed in these children, the medical profession started to take seriously the social implications of obscure and unrelated injuries.[11]

The imaging of a battered child is not limited to the extremities. A diagnosis of healing, unexplained fractures at the ends of the long bones in a child brought in because of an acute injury is a significant indication for further evaluation and investigation. Typically, new fractures at the ends of the long bones are through the metaphysis or are of the "bucket handle" type, in which fragments of bone are detached, and the periosteum is still attached (Fig. 6–20).

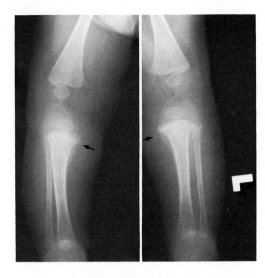

Figure 6-20

Radiographs of a 2-month-old infant who was admitted with a head injury. Child abuse was suspected, and a skeletal survey was performed. Bucket handle fractures (*arrows*) are visible at the ends of both proximal tibiae and the left fibula.

The routine projections described are those listed by Paul K. Kleinman,[12] who notes that all positive sites should be radiographed in at least two projections.[12]

Routine Projections: Anteroposterior supine chest, lateral chest; anteroposterior humeri, forearms; posteroanterior hands; anteroposterior pelvis, lateral lumbar spine, femora, tibiae, feet; anteroposterior and lateral skull.

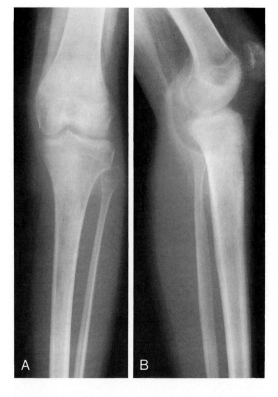

Figure 6-21

A, Anteroposterior and *B*, lateral views of the tibia and fibula in a 14-year-old male, showing bone changes in the proximal tibia consistent with osteosarcoma.

OSTEOSARCOMA

Osteosarcoma is an extremely malignant primary bone tumor. It can affect almost any part of the skeleton but is primarily found at the ends of the long bones. Although osteosarcoma can occur at any age, it is commonly found in the second decade of life, the median age being around 17 to 18 years.[13] The most common sites are those of most active epiphyseal growth, the lower end of the femur, the upper end of the tibia or fibula, and the upper end of the humerus[13] (Fig. 6–21).

The peak incidence of osteosarcoma corresponds to the peak skeletal growth of adolescence and forms in the metaphyses of the long bones. The growth potential of each long bone generally determines the frequency of tumors. Accordingly, the most common sites for osteogenic sarcoma are the femur (41.5%), the tibia (16%), and the humerus (15%).[14] The term *osteogenic* is sometimes used rather than osteosarcoma because it describes the way in which the tumor is formed; i.e., as it arises from bone, it forms bone.[14] The incidence is higher in males than in females.

The early symptom is pain, which initially may be mild, and the patient may associate (mistakenly) it with a sports-related injury. As the tumor develops, the pain becomes severe, with increasingly tender swelling over the area. Initial radiographs are routine anteroposterior and lateral views of the affected part.

Once the tumor has been diagnosed, its extent is evaluated by computed tomography, magnetic resonance imaging, and radionuclide bone scan. The latter is particularly

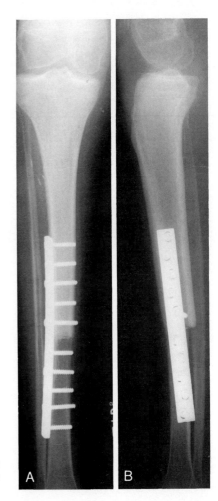

Figure 6–22

A, Anteroposterior and **B**, lateral views of the tibia and fibula following allograft of the tibia shown in Figure 6–21.

important in the detection of other bone metastases. The primary site of secondary metastases is the lung, and follow-up radiographs include posteroanterior and lateral views of the chest, followed by a computed tomography scan. To avoid amputation, an innovative procedure — allograft — is being performed, in which the diseased bone is replaced with bone from a cadaver (Fig. 6–22).

Routine Projections: Anteroposterior, oblique, and lateral views of the affected limb.

REFERENCES

1. Rang, M., Children's Fractures, J.B. Lippincott Company, Philadelphia, 1983
2. Salter, R.B., and Harris, R., Injuries involving the epiphyseal plate, Journal of Bone and Joint Surgery, 45:587–622, 1963
3. Wilkinson, R.H., Epiphyseal injuries, Applied Radiology 18(12):13–18, 1989
4. Greulich, W.W., and Pyle, S.I., Radiographic Atlas of Skeletal Development of the Hand and Wrist, 2nd ed., Stanford University Press, Stanford, CA, 1959, [Printing, 1988]
5. Reed, M.H., Ed., Pediatric Skeletal Radiology, Williams & Wilkins, Baltimore, 1992
6. Chew, F.S., Skeletal Radiology. The Bare Bones, Aspen Publications, Rockville, MD, 1989
7. Brodeur, A.E., Silberstein, M.J., and Graviss, E.R., Radiology of the Pediatric Elbow, G.K. Hall Publishers, Boston, 1981
8. Tachdjian, M.O., The Child's Foot, W.B. Saunders Company, Philadelphia, 1985
9. Oestreich, A.H., Skeletal system, in Practical Pediatric Imaging. Diagnostic Radiology of Infants and Children, 2nd ed., D.R. Kirks, Ed., Little, Brown & Company, Boston, 1991
10. Caffey, J., Multiple fractures in the long bones of children, American Journal of Radiology, 56:163–173, 1946
11. Newberger, E.H., Editor, Child Abuse, Little, Brown & Company, Boston, 1982
12. Kleinman, P.K., Diagnostic Imaging in Infant Abuse, American Journal of Radiology, 155:703–712, 1990
13. Huvos, A.G., Bone Tumors: Diagnosis, Treatment and Prognosis, W.B. Saunders Company, Philadelphia, 1979
14. Salter, R.B., Textbook of Disorders and Injuries of the Musculoskeletal System, Williams & Wilkins, Baltimore, 1984

The Spine

DEVELOPMENT

Most people are born with seven cervical, twelve thoracic, five lumbar, and five sacral vertebrae and three or four coccygeal segments. A few have one or two more or less.[1] The absence of one vertebra in one segment may be compensated by another in the adjacent section of the spine.[1]

The skeleton is of mesodermal origin, and most of its parts go through three stages of development: (1) a membranous, mesenchymal stage, (2) a cartilaginous stage, and (3) ossification, which has substages, primary and secondary.[2]

The vertebral column is formed from the embryonic notochord, which is a solid but flexible rod of cells surrounded by a membranous sheath. The notochord acts as a framework around which the mesenchymal vertebrae are formed. Chondrification (formation of the cartilaginous vertebrae) begins around the 6th week of fetal life at the cervicothoracic junction and extends caudally and cranially.[2]

Primary ossification begins around the 8th or 9th week of fetal life.[2] Ossification centers appear first in the neural arches of the cervical and thoracic regions and extend caudally and also appear in the bodies of the lower thoracic and upper lumbar vertebrae, extending both cranially and caudally. Each vertebral body is ossified from two centers, one anterior and one posterior to the degenerating notochord.[2]

At the center of each body is the centrum. During the first years of life, there is cartilage between the centrum and the neural arch, called the neurocentral synchondrosis. Bony fusion between the arches and the centrum takes place first in the upper cervical vertebrae during the 3rd year and progresses inferiorly. It is complete in the lower lumbar region by the 6th year.[2]

The odontoid process, or dens, is separated by a cartilaginous plate from the body of the axis in infants and persists until the 6th year. The tip of the dens develops a secondary ossification center at age 2 and fuses at around age 12.[2]

On radiographs of the neonate, vertebral bodies tend to appear rectangular in the thoracic region and oval in the lumbar region. A "bone within a bone" appearance, considered a growth stage, is normal for the first few months of life.[3]

Secondary centers of ossification form at the superior and inferior margins of the vertebral bodies between 8 and 10 years of age.[2] On a lateral radiograph, these appear as steplike defects or, as ossification progresses, wedge-shaped fragments and may be confused with abnormal processes by those not familiar with pediatric anatomy.[2] Other secondary ossification centers appear around puberty at the tips of the spinous processes, the transverse processes, and the articulating facets.[1] Fusion of all secondary centers is complete by age 25.

Abnormal chondrification and ossification is responsible for congenital malformation of the vertebral bodies.[2] Hemivertebrae and butterfly-shaped vertebrae may be the cause of congenital scoliosis and kyphosis. Fusion of one vertebra or more, for example, in the cervical spine, gives rise to a short neck, as in Klippel-Feil syndrome. Nonfusion of the posterior neural arch without neurologic abnormality is known as spina bifida occulta. Spina bifida with meningocele (herniation of the meninges) and spina bifida with myelomeningocele (herniation of both cord and meninges) are complex neurologic conditions with associated spine and hip deformities.[2]

The vertebral column provides support for the trunk and protection for the spinal cord. Viewed from the side in the adolescent, it has four normal curves (Fig. 7–1). The thoracic and sacral curves are concave forward and are primary curves, i.e., they are present at birth. The cervical and lumbar curves are considered secondary or compensatory curves, i.e., they are developmental. The cervical curve is lordotic and develops as an infant starts to hold up its head and sit upright. The lumbar curve is also lordotic and develops as a child starts to walk.

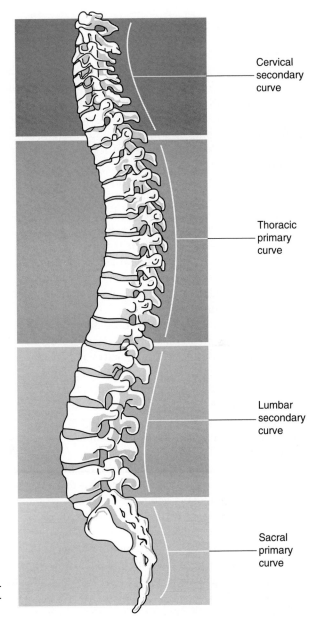

Cervical
secondary
curve

Thoracic
primary
curve

Lumbar
secondary
curve

Sacral
primary
curve

Figure 7-1
Diagram showing the four normal primary and secondary vertebral curves.

Diminished kyphosis in the thoracic spine and thoracic lordosis are abnormal. Juvenile thoracic kyphosis (Scheuermann disease) is common in adolescence, and its etiology is obscure.[4] The affected vertebrae are wedged anteriorly, disk spaces are narrowed, and irregular notches are visible on the anterosuperior aspects of the vertebral borders below the involved discs.[4]

Scoliosis is a lateral rotatory curve and not only may be due to congenital deformity but also may develop as a result of a neuromuscular disorder (such as cerebral palsy, tumor, paralysis, or trauma) or may be idiopathic (of unknown origin). Patients with congenital heart disease or Marfan syndrome may also develop scoliosis. Radiation therapy of the kidney for Wilms' tumor may cause scoliosis owing to growth retardation of the spine on the treated side.

SCOLIOSIS

Scoliosis (lateral curvature of the spine) develops for different reasons; this section addresses the most common form: adolescent idiopathic scoliosis.

Scoliosis may be nonstructural or structural. Nonstructural scoliosis is usually due to extrinsic factors such as leg shortening, hip dysplasia, tumor, or pain. The spine straightens when the patient is recumbent. In structural scoliosis, not only is there a lateral curvature but the vertebral bodies have a rotatory component (Fig. 7–2), and the spine will not straighten when the patient is supine or the spine is in forward flexion.[5]

Idiopathic scoliosis is a structural disorder and is now considered to be genetic in origin. When a diagnosis of idiopathic scoliosis is made in a mother or daughter, other siblings at the age of risk should be evaluated.[6] Mild curves are common in young children and are rarely progressive, but once a curve has progressed beyond 30 degrees in a child whose skeletal growth is not completed, progression is almost inevitable.[5]

Idiopathic scoliosis is categorized by age group: infantile (from birth to age 3), juvenile (ages 3 to 10), and adolescent (over age 10). Idiopathic scoliosis is the most common form of lateral curvature of the spine, accounting for 65% of cases in adolescents with structural scoliosis.[5]

Scoliosis may be first noticed by parents as a postural deformity or detected in a school screening program. School screening programs are mandatory in approximately one-third of schools in the United States and are conducted on students in fifth to ninth grades.[4] The literature, while stressing the positive aspects of diagnosing scoliosis early, reflects concern that many children with mild, nonprogressive curves undergo needless tests and referrals, including unnecessary radiographic examinations. Wenger and Rang[6] state that in school screening programs, no more than about 5 patients in 100 should be referred for further evaluation. With trained, experienced evaluators, no more than 3 in 100 need be referred.

In the past, when a child had been diagnosed with scoliosis, the progression of the curve was monitored at 6-month intervals by radiographing the spine with the patient lying, standing, bending, and sometimes in traction. Considering the slower speeds of screen/film combinations used 25 years ago, the number of radiographs taken, and radiation exposure, the radiation dose for the patient was considerably higher than it is today. Because scoliosis is particularly prevalent in young adolescent girls, and radiographs were taken with the patient facing the x-ray tube as well as lateral to the tube, the breasts, without lead protection, received the highest (skin entrance) dose. As discussed in the chapter on radiation protection, research has shown an increase in breast cancer in women whose breasts were exposed to x-radiation during adolescence.[7]

Screening for scoliosis includes assessing shoulder height, pelvic asymmetry, and scapular and flank asymmetry. In London in 1882, W. Adams proposed the forward bending test to assess rib asymmetry, as scoliosis is not always seen when a patient is standing[6] (Fig. 7–3). A scoliometer placed on the patient's back measures the angle of trunk rotation. Common curve patterns are right thoracic, left lumbar, left thoracolumbar, and double right thoracic and left lumbar.

If screening detects a mild structural curve, progression is monitored during the period of most rapid growth, which extends through puberty. A bone-age radiograph of the left hand and wrist is taken to assess skeletal maturity.

Curve progression can be monitored by methods other than exposing patients to ionizing radiation. The alternatives do not replace the accuracy of the radiographic measurement of scoliosis but may be efficacious and inexpensive in detecting changes in mild idiopathic curves. Two of these alternatives are moire topography and the Integrated Shape Investigation System (ISIS). In their article on the management of

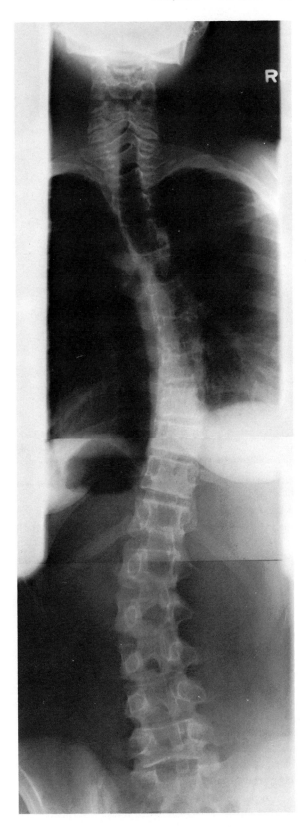

Figure 7-2
Standing view of the spine, C1–S2 (view from the back), showing scoliosis with a right thoracic and left lumbar curve with a rotary component in the upper lumbar vertebrae.

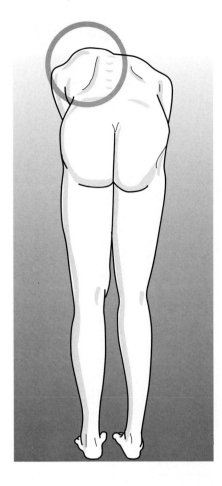

Figure 7-3

Adams forward bending test, showing rib hump asymmetry indicative of thoracolumbar scoliosis.

adolescent scoliosis, Casella and Hall state that for mild curves "a roentgenogram is necessary only if there is a significant change in the moire pattern or ISIS contour."[5]

Statistically, we are radiographing fewer patients for scoliosis at Children's Hospital, and a brief description of the surface measurement techniques we use shows how they can be used as a substitute for radiography.

MOIRÉ TOPOGRAPHY

Moiré contour pattern is an optical effect used to provide a topographic outline of the body. The patient stands behind a grid of equally spaced horizontal or vertical lines illuminated by a point light source.[8] When viewed through the grid, the lines and shadows appear as a series of points of interference, which are then viewed as contour lines on the patient. These contour lines create a moiré pattern (similar to that sometimes seen in silk fabric) on the patient's back. For accurate representation of surface contours, a fixed distance between the light source and the point of view (in this case a photographic camera) must be maintained. The light source and the camera must be in the same parallel plane as the grid.[8]

A person with a straight spine will have almost symmetrical contour patterns. The radiograph of a person with spinal curvature shows asymmetrical shadow patterns when the left side of the back is compared with the right because of the spine's tendency to rotate on its axis as it curves laterally[8] (Fig. 7-4).

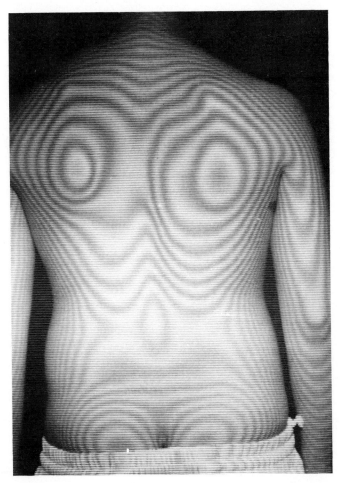

Figure 7–4
Asymmetrical moiré contour pattern (view from the back), showing right rib hump indicative of a left thoracic curve.

INTEGRATED SHAPE INVESTIGATION SYSTEM

The ISIS is an automated optical stereophotogrammetric system that quantifies the shape of the back in three dimensions.[9] The system produces an outline of the back in three planes and, because positioning is repeatable, monitors changes that occur. The ISIS consists of a video camera and a light source mounted on a scanning unit. The projector produces a horizontal band of light that scans the patient's back from top to bottom using a rotating mirror controlled by a computer console.[9]

The patient stands with the back to the light source and camera. Matte black stickers about 1 inch square are placed at evenly spaced intervals on the spinous processes. The uppermost one is at the C7–T1 level, and the two lowest, one on each side, are at the level of the posterior superior iliac spines (PSISs). The light band gives the computer the upper and lower landmarks before scanning begins. Scan time is about 2 seconds.

The computer screen first shows a body outline, from which transverse sections are computed, rather like slicing a loaf of bread. These sections show the differences in the height of the back at various levels and the rotational effect of the scoliosis. Lateral

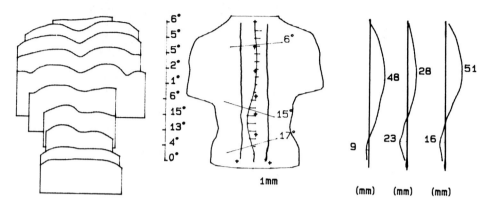

Figure 7–5
Integrated shape investigation system (ISIS) computerized topographic printout showing (from left to right) transverse, posteroanterior, and three sagittal profiles.

asymmetry is then shown on the body outline. The computed measurements are similar to Cobb angle measurements. These measurements are followed by three sagittal profiles comparing kyphotic and lordotic points. A printout, available within about 5 minutes, gives a visual sense of the shape of the patient's back (Fig. 7–5).

SCOLIOMETER

The scoliometer, which looks a little like a level, is a simple scale used for measuring the angle of trunk rotation. The patient is asked to bend forward, and the scale is placed straddling the spinous processes at the areas of greatest asymmetry. The scale is marked in 1-degree intervals on each side of a central zero. The mark where the bubble rests is the degree of rotation. A curve will be investigated further if the angle of rotation is greater than 5 degrees. The scoliometer is used by many pediatric orthopedic surgeons and is inexpensive, practical, and readily available.

RADIOGRAPHIC TECHNIQUE

Whereas the methods described previously are for evaluating curve progression, radiographs are necessary to evaluate structural anatomy and deformity. Fortunately, from the perspective of radiation dose, the "scoliosis series" developed many years ago, consisting of multiple views, is no longer necessary. The most common request at Children's Hospital is to obtain one erect view (posteroanterior projection) of the complete spine from C1 to the level of the anterior superior iliac spine (ASIS) on a 36-inch film (Fig. 7–6). The dose to the growing breast tissues is greatly reduced when the patient faces the cassette in the posteroanterior projection. An erect lateral projection on the same size film may also be requested on a first examination when the patient has pain or a deformity or before surgery (Fig. 7–7).

The Cobb method is most widely used by radiologists and orthopedic surgeons to measure the scoliosis curve on a posteroanterior radiograph. A sharp pencil, a rule, and a protractor are needed for calculating the measurements. A line is drawn along the superior border of the upper-end vertebra. This is the highest vertebra at which the

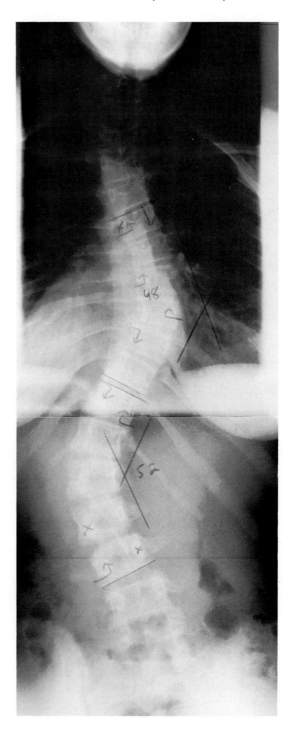

Figure 7–6

Standing posteroanterior view of the spine, from the back, showing right thoracic and left lumbar curves. Note the Cobb angle measurements.

superior border is inclined toward the thoracic concavity. A second line is drawn along the inferior border of the transitional vertebra. This is the lowest vertebra at which the inferior border is inclined toward the thoracic concavity and the highest vertebra inclined toward the lumbar concavity. A perpendicular line is then drawn from each of these lines; the Cobb angle is the point at which they intersect[10] (Fig. 7–8). Wenger states that as much as a 5-degree interexaminer error can occur in these measurements;

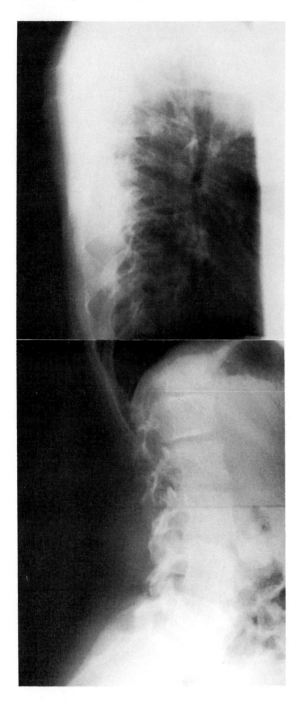

Figure 7-7
Standing lateral view of the spine shown in Figure 7-6. Note the breast shielding.

this should be explained to parents and patients who are already concerned about changes in the curve and the possibility of corrective surgery.[6]

Right and left bending radiographs may be requested before surgery to assess the natural ability of the spine to correct curvature and vertebral rotation. The patient is supine for these radiographs and bends the trunk first to one side and then the other. It is important that while maintaining the bending position, the patient keep the shoulders and pelvis flat and in contact with the table. It usually takes two films (14 by

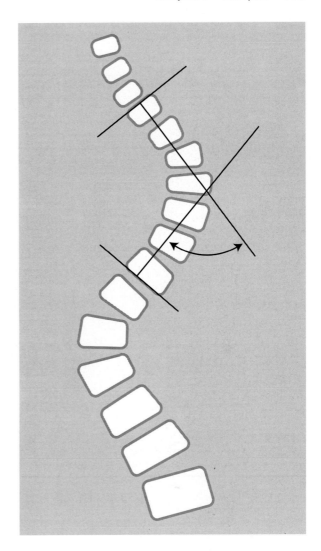

Figure 7–8
The Cobb method of measuring
scoliosis.

17 inches) to cover the complete spine on each bend. The patient should not move
between the two exposures of the bend on the same side (Fig. 7–9).

Routine Projections: On the initial examination, posteroanterior standing spine
from C1 to the level of the ASIS on a 36-inch cassette at a 72-inch SID. Lateral
view on request. On a preoperative examination, posteroanterior, lateral, right
and left bending views.

Technical Considerations: A wedge filter should be used to even the density
between the cervical, thoracic, and lumbar spines. On the posteroanterior projection,
the breasts receive the exit rather than the skin entrance radiation dose. A wedge
filter/breast shield assembly similar to the one described in Chapter 14 can be used. A
1200-speed screen/film system is recommended. This is a high-contrast system and
appears grainy owing to quantum mottle, but when spinal curvature rather than bone

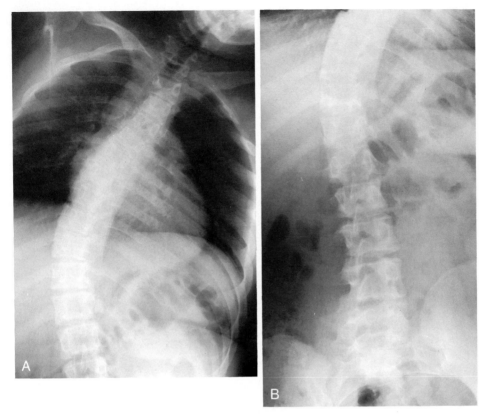

Figure 7-9

A and *B*, Overlapping projections to cover the whole spine, with the patient supine and bending to the left, to evaluate curve reduction. Straightening of the upper thoracic curvature is incomplete.

detail is being evaluated, the resulting radiographs are satisfactory at a lower radiation dose.

To assess the exposure, measure the patient from front to back, at the nipple line in a male and just under the breasts in a female. The skin entrance radiation dose for a posteroanterior projection at Children's Hospital is estimated at 48 mR on a patient measuring 17 to 20 cm, using an exposure technique of 75 kVp and 20 mAs. The exit dose to the breasts without lead shielding is 1 to 2 mrad. The iliac crests and the rib cage should be included on the initial study, as orthopedic surgeons are usually interested in evaluating rib deformity and the trunk as a whole, not just the vertebral column.

TREATMENT

Because patients are frequently radiographed in a brace, both during and after spinal surgery, a brief overview of current treatment practices seems appropriate. For many years, various types of braces have been used to try to correct a curve or halt the progression of a curve. The brace that first effectively managed curve control was the Milwaukee brace. It was developed by Blount and Schmidt in the 1950's.[6] The superstructure was metal and the padding and straps were leather. The metal superstructure extended to the base of the skull posteriorly and to the chin anteriorly. Many teenagers believed that a social stigma was attached to wearing such a brace; consequently, the

Milwaukee brace, which was visible when worn as prescribed, was considered unsightly. The brace was successful, but many young patients objected to wearing it.

In the 1970's, the Boston Bracing System (BBS) developed by Hall and Miller eliminated the superstructure.[6] Variations of the BBS are referred to as either low-profile or thoracolumbar-sacral orthoses.[5] The BBS—a prefabricated lightweight brace of polypropylene with a soft inner lining of polyethylene—is customized to fit the individual patient (Fig. 7–10). The brace fits under the arms, has no protruding metal neck piece, and can be worn under clothing; thus, it is potentially more acceptable to teenagers.

Bracing is used for moderate curves to prevent the progression of scoliosis and thus avoid surgery and for more severe curves in younger patients, with the hope of delaying surgery until the child has finished growing. Originally, a brace was to be worn 23 out of 24 hours and removed only when bathing.[5] Today at Children's Hospital patients are initially instructed to wear the brace 22 to 24 hours a day. After 6 to 9 months, if the curve is holding, they can reduce the time they wear it to 18 hours a day. Patients decide when to take off their brace, and many remove it for after-school activities.

The spine is checked radiographically both in and out of the brace. The first in-brace radiograph is taken at 3 to 4 weeks to see if in-brace correction is being achieved (the ideal is 50% improvement in the curve) and then at 4-month intervals. The out-of-brace radiographs are taken to see if a curve is holding. Patients typically wear a brace until they have finished growing. Technically, there is no need to increase the exposure for radiographs taken in these plastic braces.

SURGICAL INTERVENTION AND INSTRUMENTATION

Indications for corrective surgical treatment of scoliosis include prevention of back pain, possible cardiopulmonary complications, and cosmetic reasons. Earlier proce-

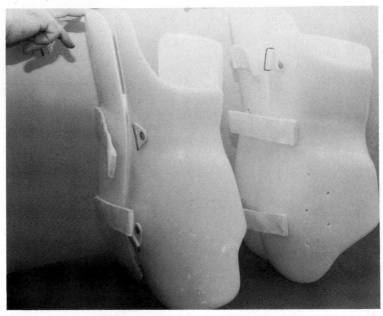

Figure 7–10
Customized polyethylene Boston braces.

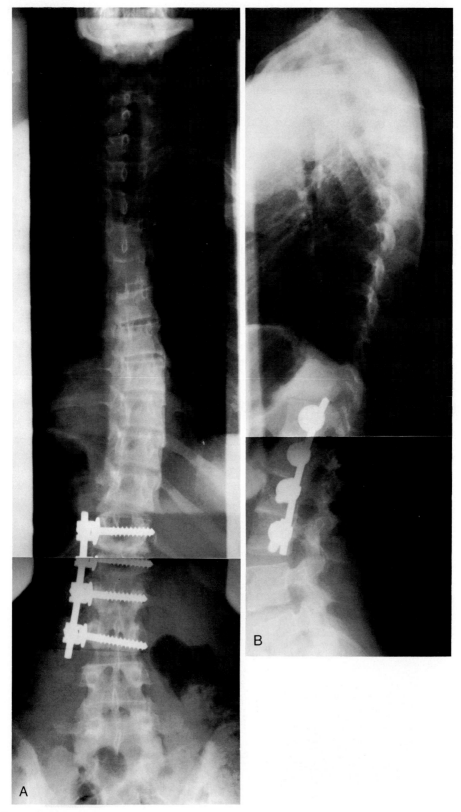

Figure 7–11

The Texas Scottish Rite Hospital instrumentation system is an anterior segmental approach to improving the stability of the spine. **A**, Posteroanterior view. **B**, Lateral view.

dures involved extensive correction using, for example, the Risser turnbuckle cast before spinal fusion. After surgery, patients spent many months in a full-body plaster cast.

In the 1960's, the Harrington instrumentation method improved stability and correctability by attaching distraction-and-compression stainless steel rods to the spine.[6] This method effectively "jacked up" the spine, and although greater stability was achieved, patients still had to wear a full-body cast for a long time after surgery. Another type of instrumentation is the anterior segmental approach. In the Dwyer method, screws are placed through the sides of the vertebral bodies, and correction is achieved by looping and tightening titanium cable around the heads of the screws. Zielke, from Germany, further modified this system.[6] Another anterior segmental approach we use at Children's Hospital is the Texas Scottish Rite Hospital system (Fig. 7–11).

In the 1970's, Eduardo Luque of Mexico developed a method of wiring rods to the spine for greater stability.[6] This method is used mainly for paralytic curves and not for idiopathic scoliosis because of the risk of neurologic complications due to the sublaminar position of the wires (Fig. 7–12).

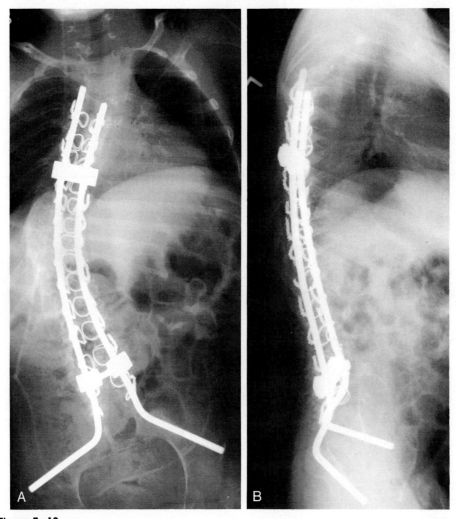

Figure 7–12

Luque instrumentation in a patient with one long paralytic curve. **A,** Anteroposterior view. **B,** Lateral view.

In the 1980's, two Frenchman, Cotrel and Dubousset, developed an instrumentation system that not only straightened the curves but also corrected the vertebral rotation.[6] The Cotrel-Dubousset system uses two rods (7 mm in diameter) and multiple hooks, which can face either cranially or caudally, correcting the scoliosis in three dimensions (Fig. 7–13). The advantage of this instrumentation is that the multiple attachment sites make it very stable. Patients go home a week after surgery and usually do not require postoperative immobilization.

In most cases, the goal of spinal instrumentation is to provide both correction and

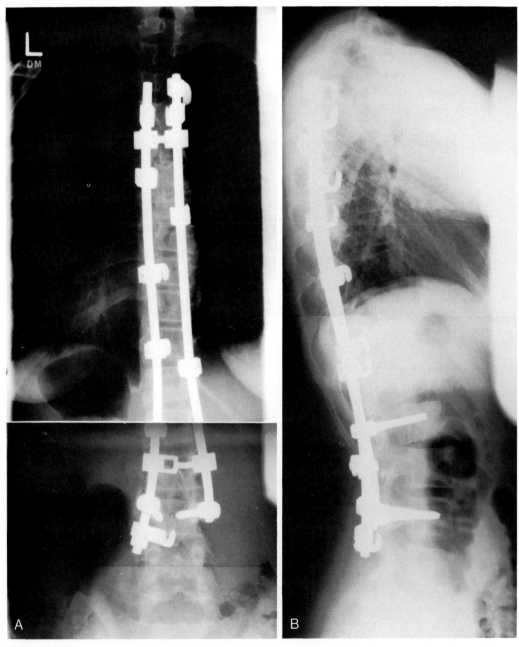

Figure 7–13

Cotrel-Dubousset instrumentation, showing correction in the patient shown in Figures 7–6 and 7–7. **A**, Posteroanterior view. **B**, Lateral view.

immobilization.[11] The choice of treatment and type of instrumentation is dependent upon the type of deformity, the pathologic process causing it, the age of the child, whether there will be continued growth, and the physical and psychological consequences of either prolonged nonsurgical or surgical treatment.[11]

> **Routine Projections:** Follow-up after instrumentation; posteroanterior and lateral standing spine from C1 to the level of the ASIS on a 36-inch cassette at a 72-inch SID. Use wedge filter and breast shields.

CERVICAL SPINE TRAUMA

Cervical spine injuries are less common in infants and children than in adolescents and adults. Patients with cervical spine injuries fall into two categories: those who can walk and move their necks and those who cannot walk and are unconscious.[12] Cervical spine injuries tend to involve the upper levels of the cervical spine (C1–C3) in infants and are more common in levels C3–C7 in older children.[12]

A high-quality radiograph is essential for the radiologist to differentiate the normal from the abnormal on a plain radiograph, and it is important to be able to visualize all seven cervical vertebrae. Cervical spine injuries range from minimal soft tissue and ligamentous injury to a complete fracture-dislocation with spinal cord injury.[12] The intervertebral disc spaces of the cervical vertebrae in normal patients are equal in height. Any discrepancy raises the possibility of a longitudinal ligament injury and suggests instability.[12] The cervical spine develops a normal lordotic curve after infancy but may appear straight on a radiograph after a trauma because of muscle spasm.

Odontoid fractures may be seen in infants and young children (Fig. 7–14). The fracture is usually through the cartilaginous area, which is the synchondrosis between the dens and the body.[12] Injury to the upper cervical spine is frequently associated with

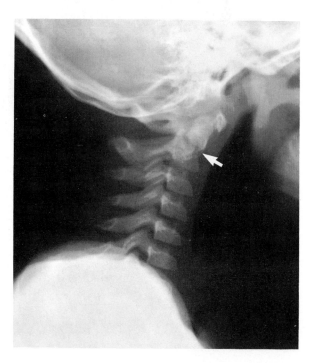

Figure 7–14

Lateral view of the cervical spine of a 3-year-old child, showing an odontoid fracture (*arrow*), with moderate anterior displacement.

head trauma. Computed tomography may be used to confirm or identify fractures, but decisions concerning the stability of an injury are based on plain radiographs.[12]

The lateral view of the cervical spine is considered the most informative. The view must be true lateral for the radiologist to evaluate the soft tissues, disc spaces, vertebral bodies, apophyseal joints, neural arches, and C1–dens distance. Extreme care must always be taken when radiographing the cervical spine after an injury to avoid damaging the spinal cord. The patient's head and neck should be immobilized in the emergency room, if not at the site of the injury. Because a young child's head is disproportionately larger than the shoulders, immobilizing the cervical spine should be approached differently than for an adult. Placing a child directly onto a backboard thrusts the head and neck forward. To ensure that the cervical spine is immobilized in line with the body, the shoulders and trunk should be elevated with padding. The emergency room staff at Children's Hospital recommends using a cervical collar (of the appropriate size) to stabilize the spine and, at the same time, to maintain an open airway. The child is then secured to a backboard with straps; any open spaces should be padded with towels and blankets to prevent movement.

A lateral projection is taken first; this can be done with the patient on the stretcher. Care must be taken not to move the patient (Fig. 7–15A). After this radiograph has been evaluated and the spine judged to be stable, an anteroposterior projection (Fig. 7–15B) and an anteroposterior projection through the open mouth of the odontoid process may be taken (Fig. 7–15C). The latter is not always possible for a young child and is impossible for an infant. Lateral flexion and extension views may be requested, depending on the injury and the stability of the spine.

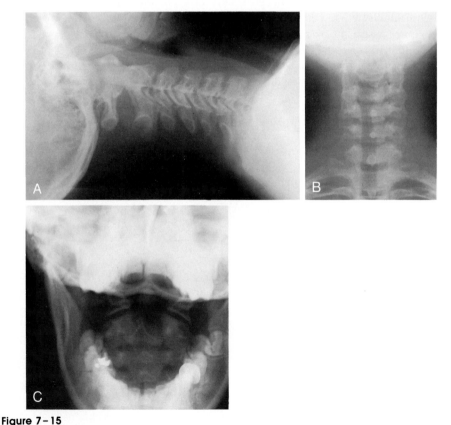

Figure 7–15

A, Lateral cervical spine of a 13-year-old child (horizontal ray lateral view). **B**, Anteroposterior view. **C**, Open-mouth view (to show C1–C2).

It is important to remember that a spinal cord injury can be present without radiographic abnormality. Thus, extreme care must always be taken when positioning or moving patients after a cervical spine injury.

Routine Projections: Lateral view first, for evaluation by a radiologist or emergency room physician, followed by anteroposterior and anteroposterior of the odontoid process open through the mouth if the child is able to cooperate.

CERVICAL SPINE IN DOWN SYNDROME

Down syndrome, also termed trisomy 21 syndrome (there is an extra chromosome, number 21), occurs in approximately 1 of 1,000 live births.[13] Children with this syndrome have multiple congenital problems, including spinal abnormalities. Of these children, 6% have an abnormality of the transverse ligament, which passes behind the odontoid process or dens, holding it in place.[2] The abnormality results from laxity, malformation, or aplasia, and there is a risk of atlantoaxial subluxation in 10% to 30% of patients with this disorder.[2]

To check instability, the distance between the atlas and the dens is measured from the posteroinferior aspect of the anterior arch of the atlas to the anterior border of the dens.[3] In the neutral position, the atlas–dens distance is usually less than 3 mm. This distance may be increased in patients with Down syndrome, with possible subluxation leading to injury of the spinal cord. A radiograph demonstrating the atlantoaxial articulation is recommended for patients at 5 years of age, particularly those interested in participating in sports activities.[13] The Special Olympics Committee has a policy of screening all patients with Down syndrome for atlantoaxial subluxation.[14]

At Children's Hospital, we use a cervical scale to aid in the accurate measurement of the atlas–dens space. The scale consists of metal tines 1 mm wide embedded in acrylic, with gaps 1 mm wide between the tines.[14] The scale is attached to a Velcro strap that is placed around the patient's neck like a collar. The scale is then on the same plane as the cervical spine, avoiding the inaccuracies of measurement related to magnification. A metal pin in the acrylic in the front of the scale is used as an indicator that the spine is at right angles to the x-ray beam and that there is no obliquity.[14]

Routine Projections: Lateral, in flexion and extension (Fig. 7–16).

LUMBAR SPINE SPONDYLOLYSIS AND SPONDYLOLISTHESIS

Spondylolysis is descriptive of a bony defect of the pars interarticularis that most commonly affects the fifth lumbar vertebra. It is found in 3% to 10% of the general population, is more common in males than in females, and is rarely seen in children under 5 years of age.[4]

The origin of these defects is debatable but is thought to be an acute or stress fracture of the immature pars.[4] The onset of symptoms tends to coincide with puberty, when a growth spurt occurs, and the symptoms may occur as a result of repetitive stress rather than an acute injury.[6] Patients have a postural deformity mimicking scoliosis and have an abnormal gait or tight hamstrings rather than low back pain.[6]

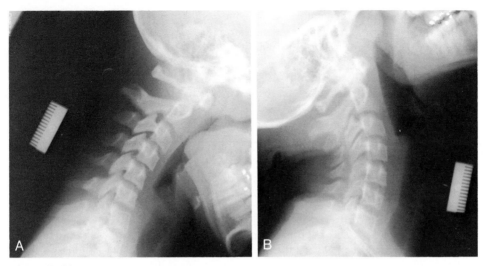

Figure 7–16
A, Flexion and **B**, extension views of the cervical spine with a scale in place.

Diagnosis is often made after trauma and when fractures through the pars interarticularis are seen radiographically. Bilateral defects in the pars and/or fracture may lead to spondylolisthesis, a forward slip of one vertebra on top of another — in Figure 7–17, of L5 on S1.[4] Some occupations that involve athletics and dancing may cause an increase in the incidence of spondylolisthesis in those genetically disposed to this condition.[4] Spondylolisthesis can occur independent of spondylolysis, with elongation of the pars interarticularis.

As in adults, the pars interarticularis is best seen on the oblique radiographs, where the neck of the "Scottie dog" configuration shows the pars, the bony mass between the articular facets.

When the radiographic examination is negative, bone scintigraphy with single photon emission computed tomography (SPECT) is recommended. SPECT shows increased activity in the pars even before the development of a true stress fracture (see Chapter 12). Computed tomography is useful to provide better anatomic definition of the pars defect and the degree of spondylolisthesis present.[15]

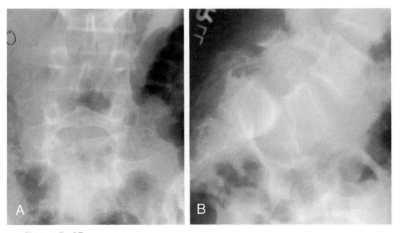

Figure 7–17
Spondylolisthesis of L5 on S1. **A**, Anteroposterior view. **B**, Lateral view.

Routine Projections: Anteroposterior, lateral, both oblique views, and a cone down of L4, L5, and sacrum to demonstrate the lumbosacral kyphosis.

Technical Considerations: A 400-speed screen/film system gives good resolution for the lowest radiation dose.

REFERENCES

1. Moore, K.L., The Developing Human, W.B. Saunders Company, Philadelphia, 1988
2. Starshak, R.J., Wells, S. J.R., Sty, J.R., and Gregg, D.C., Diagnostic Imaging of Infants and Children, Vol. 2, Aspen Publications, Gaithersburg, MD, 1992
3. Sprenger, E.C., and Ball, W.S., Jr., Spine and contents, in Practical Pediatric Imaging: Diagnostic Radiology of Infants and Children, 2nd ed., pp. 193–261, D.R. Kirks, Ed., Little, Brown & Company, Boston, 1991
4. MacPherson, R.I., Genez, B., Spine, in Pediatric Skeletal Radiology, M.H. Reed, Ed., Williams & Wilkins, Baltimore, 1992
5. Cassella, M.C., and Hall, J.E., Current treatment approaches in the nonoperative and operative management of adolescent idiopathic scoliosis, Physical Therapy, 71(12):897–909, 1991
6. Wenger, D.R., and Rang, M., The Art and Practice of Children's Orthopedics, Raven Press, New York, 1993
7. Miller, A.B., Howe, G.R., Sherman, G.J., et al., Mortality from breast cancer after irradiation during fluoroscopic examinations in patients being treated for tuberculosis, New England Journal of Medicine, 321(19):1285–1289, 1989
8. Koepfler, J.W., Moire topography in medicine, Journal of Biological Photography, 51(1):3–10, 1983
9. Turner Smith, A.R., Shannon, T.M.L., Houghton, G.R., et al, Assessing idiopathic scoliosis using a surface measurement technique, Surgical Rounds for Orthopedics, —(June):52–59, 1988
10. Cobb, J.R., Outline for the Study of Scoliosis: Instructional Course Lectures, The American Academy of Orthopedic Surgeons, J.W. Edwards Company, Ann Arbor, MI, 5:261–275, 1948
11. Emans, J.B., Instrumentation for spinal deformities in children, Orthopedic Surgery, 2(2):65–90, 1991
12. Swischuk, L., Emergency Radiology of the Acutely Ill or Injured Child, 2nd ed., Williams & Wilkins, Baltimore, 1986
13. Swaiman, K.F., Pediatric Neurology. Principles and Practice, C.V. Mosby Company, St. Louis, 1989
14. Singer, S.J., Rubin, I.L., and Strauss, K.J., Atlantoaxial distance with Down's syndrome: Standards of measurement, Radiology, 164(September):871–872, 1987
15. Bellah, R.D., Summerville, D.A., Treves, S.T., et al., Low back pain in adolescent athletes: Detection of stress injury to the pars interarticularis with SPECT, Radiology, 180:509–512, 1991

The Pelvis and Hips

DEVELOPMENT

The bones of the pelvis, sacrum, ilium, ischium, and pubis are formed in utero from cartilage. The ilium begins to ossify at 8 fetal weeks, the ischium at 16 weeks, and the pubis at 18 to 29 weeks.[1] At birth there is still wide separation by cartilage between the ossified parts of the bones, which radiographically appear unconnected because the cartilage radiographically blends in with the other soft tissues (Fig. 8–1).

The acetabulum, which is formed by the ilium, ischium, and pubis, is also cartilage at birth and is a well-developed concavity in a normal infant. The Y-shaped triradiate cartilage separating these bones persists until it ossifies between ages 13 and 15 years.[1] The femoral head is not seen radiographically until it starts to ossify between ages 3 to 6 months. Fusion of the femoral head epiphysis occurs between ages 14 and 17 years.[1]

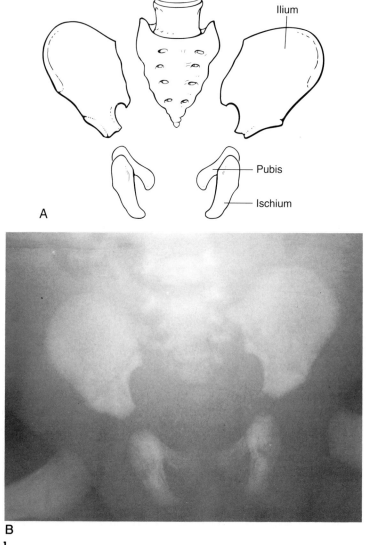

Figure 8–1

A, Diagram and **B**, radiograph of the pelvis of a newborn, showing separation between the ilium, ischium, and pubis.

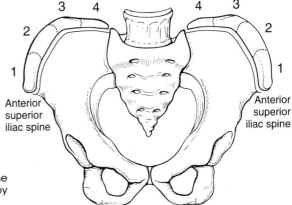

Figure 8–2

Diagram showing maturation of the iliac apophysis, as described by Risser in 1958.

The appearance of the epiphyses and apophyses varies not only with age but also with gender, as female skeletal maturation is generally more advanced than that of males.

The apophyseal ossification center for the greater trochanter appears at age 5 years and fuses in girls at age 14 years and in boys at age 17 years.[1] The lesser trochanter (in males) appears between ages 12 and 16 years, the ischial tuberosity at ages 16 to 19 years, and the iliac crest at ages 14 to 16 years.[1] The iliac crest, usually the last to fuse, is complete by age 2 years.

The iliac crest excursion of ossification, used as a skeletal maturation guideline, was described by Risser in 1958.[2] The apophysis is divided into four quarters, starting at the anterior superior iliac spine (ASIS). Risser 1 is 25%, Risser 2 is 50%, Risser 3 is 75%, and Risser 4 is complete excursion[2,3] (Fig. 8–2). When the apophysis fuses with the body of the ilium, it is graded Risser 5.

Recognition of skeletal maturation is important, as many diseases and conditions related to childhood are reflected by changes in growth patterns. Avulsion fractures of incompletely fused apophyses are common, as are fractures or slips of the physes, the weaker parts of a growing skeleton.

RADIOGRAPHIC TECHNIQUE

Both hips should be routinely radiographed as the initial examination. Bilateral radiographs are helpful to compare the affected side with the healthy hip, and developmental dysplasia of the hip (DDH), Legg-Calvé-Perthes disease, and slipped capital femoral epiphysis (SCFE) frequently affect both hips. For follow-up after treatment, radiographs of only the affected hip may be necessary.

> **Technical Considerations:** A 400-speed screen/film system gives satisfactory detail for the lowest radiation dose.

DEVELOPMENTAL DYSPLASIA OF THE HIP

In 1991 the Pediatric Orthopedic Society of North America replaced the term *congenital dislocation of the hip* (CDH) with *developmental dysplasia of the hip* (DDH).[1] The predisposition to this condition may arise in utero, depending on the position of the fetus. In the normal intrauterine position, the hips are flexed so that the femoral head maintains its proper position in the acetabulum.[1] Dislocation may occur as a result of the knees' being extended, as occurs in some breech presentations. It may also occur because of the way in which a fetus is lying in utero. When the left hip in utero is more restricted in its movement than the right, a unilateral left-sided dislocation can result.[1]

Not all factors contributing to DDH are known, and a combination of joint laxity, a shallow acetabulum, intrauterine position, and hormonal influences may contribute to hip instability in the newborn.[3] It is a common abnormality—the incidence is 1.5 to 10 per 1,000 live births.[4] Girls are affected five times more often than boys.[5] The left hip is affected more often than the right, and 5% to 20% of cases are bilateral.[4] A clinical diagnosis is made when there is partial or complete displacement of the femoral head from the acetabulum as the femur is abducted.[1] In severe cases the femoral head will dislocate spontaneously.[4]

Radiographic findings may be subtle in a newborn, and a normal radiograph of the hips does not exclude a diagnosis of DDH. Because the femoral head is not ossified at birth, its position is assessed on a radiograph by the orientation of the proximal femoral metaphysis with respect to the pelvis.[4] Later, ossification of the femoral head may be delayed because of displacement and a shallow acetabulum (Fig. 8–3).

There are various methods of measuring the angle of the acetabular roof and the degree of dislocation before ossification of the femoral head. One method described by Hilgenreiner in 1925 involves measuring the angle between the sloping roof of the acetabulum and a horizontal line drawn through the Y cartilages.[5] This horizontal line is known as the Y-Y line (Fig. 8–4). Lines drawn from the Y-Y line to the middle of the superior aspect of the femoral shafts measure lateral displacement.[5]

The best radiographic method of demonstrating DDH has always been controversial. Many pediatricians say that DDH can be diagnosed by clinical examination rather than by the use of ionizing radiation. Radiographically, it is difficult to maintain an infant's pelvis flat on an x-ray table for a true anteroposterior projection of the hips. Other radiographic positions used to diagnose DDH include the frog-leg lateral and the von Rosen, first described by Andrén and von Rosen of Sweden in 1958.[6] Because the frog-leg lateral is also the treatment position, many radiologists think that using this position tends to reduce the dislocation of an unstable hip, rather than demonstrate it radiographically.

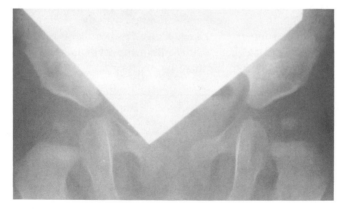

Figure 8–3
Femoral head ossification is slightly smaller on the right than on the left, suggesting earlier subluxation or dislocation.

R   L

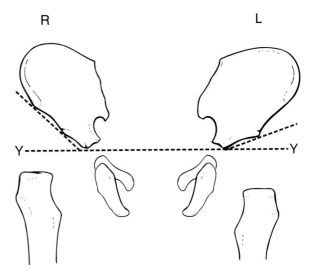

Figure 8–4
Hilgenreiner method of measuring the angle between the roof of the acetabulum and a horizontal line drawn through the Y cartilages before ossification of the femoral head occurs. The normal acetabular angle is on the left; the abnormal acetabular angle is on the right, showing lateral displacement of the right femur.

The von Rosen technique involves abducting the legs 45 degrees and positioning the hips in full internal rotation. The hip or hips tend to dislocate in this position if there is joint instability. The problem lies in maintaining the hips and the legs equidistant and in a similar position for comparison purposes. Houston maintains that this view is reliable in neonates only if they are positioned by an experienced pediatric radiologist or orthopedic surgeon.[1]

The imaging procedure of choice in infants under 1 year is ultrasonography. From birth to 6 months, ultrasonography is considered more accurate than radiography and avoids the use of ionizing radiation. The procedure, however, must be performed by an experienced ultrasonographer to ensure that an accurate diagnosis is made. At Children's Hospital we perform approximately 1,100 ultrasound examinations per year on infants with a possible diagnosis of DDH. Ultrasonography is also used to follow an infant being treated for DDH, although radiographs may be taken to confirm placement of the femoral head at ages 6 and 12 months.[1]

Treatment depends on the diagnosis and when the diagnosis is made. A subluxatable hip in a neonate may stabilize within a few weeks if immobilized in abduction and flexion by double or triple diapering.[7] If a hip is dislocated or dislocatable, immobilization and reduction may be done with a harness. One commonly used harness was developed by Pavlik, a Czechoslovakian orthopedic surgeon, in the 1950's.[7] It is important when taking follow-up radiographs of the hips out of a brace or harness not to extend the infant's legs, as this could jeopardize the stability of the hip.

Positive-contrast hip arthrography may be performed in the operating room by orthopedic surgeons in more complex cases. Computed tomography may be used as follow-up after reduction, with the patient in a spica cast (Fig. 8–5).

Routine Projections: From birth to 6 months, initially, anteroposterior and von Rosen (preferably positioned by a physician). Over age 6 months and for follow-up examinations, anteroposterior and/or frog-leg lateral. Out of harness follow-up examination, one view of the hips in 45 degrees of flexion and 45 degrees of abduction. Use gonadal shielding except on the initial radiograph. Care should be taken not to obscure the acetabulum.

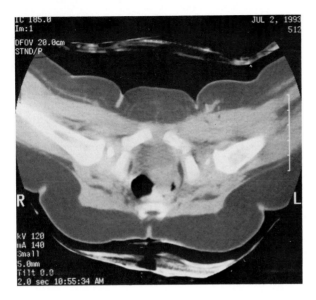

Figure 8–5
Computed tomography scan showing both hips in a spica cast. The left dislocation after reduction shows the femoral head within the acetabulum. Note that the left femoral ossification center is smaller.

Ultrasonography up to 6 months of age is considered more accurate than radiography for patients in assessing the depth of the acetabulum and the cartilaginous femoral head. It is equally accurate in assessing the slope of the acetabulum and the degree of instability.[4] Real-time ultrasonography is performed in the transverse and coronal planes. Figure 8–6 shows a normal hip and a hip with a posterolateral displacement of the femoral head.

LEGG-CALVÉ-PERTHES DISEASE

Considered idiopathic, Legg-Calvé-Perthes disease (referred to as Perthes disease) affects children between 3 and 12 years of age but is diagnosed most frequently in children between 5 and 8 years of age.[8] The disease is common in young Caucasian

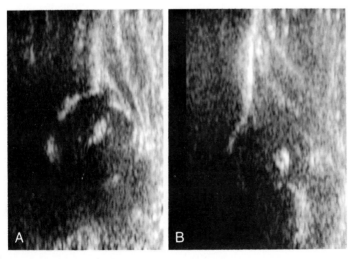

Figure 8–6
A, Ultrasound showing normal alignment. *B*, Ultrasound showing posterolateral displacement of the femoral head.

males and uncommon among Blacks. The male-female ratio is 4 : 1.[8] The disease affects either hip and it may be bilateral, but usually not simultaneously.[4] The condition may also be referred to as avascular necrosis because it is a lack of blood supply to the femoral head that prevents normal growth. The incident that triggers interruption of blood supply to all or part of the femoral epiphysis is not known.[3] The femoral epiphysis of the affected hip appears smaller than normal on a radiograph.

The major blood supply to the femoral head arises from the superior and inferior retinacular arteries, which are branches of the medial circumflex femoral artery.[4] Branches of the lateral circumflex femoral artery supply blood to the greater trochanter, the anterior aspect of the femoral neck, and a small segment of the uppermost epiphysis.[4] Because a transitional stage of development occurs between ages 4 and 7 years, when the blood supply is particularly vulnerable, it may be a minor or repeat trauma that produces the ischemia.[3] Children who have Perthes disease are short for their age, and their skeletal age may be 2 to 3 years behind their chronological age. Bone age is ascertained from a radiograph of the left hand and wrist. Current theory is that a child may have a genetic predisposition to Perthes disease.

There are several phases in Perthes disease; in the initial phase, there is vascular occlusion with bone death.[4] Because radiographically there is no difference between living bone and dead bone, radiographs may appear normal. In the next phase there is revascularization, growth impairment, and pathologic subchondral fractures through the necrotic portion of the bone.[4] Radiographs show a smaller than normal epiphysis and increased bone density. In the later stages, there is resorption of dead bone and growth of new bone.

Radiographic findings in Perthes disease include soft-tissue swelling along the lateral aspect of the joint, changes in the proximal femoral ossification center, subchondral fracture, flattening of the femoral head, and a decrease in the size of the ossification center[4] (Fig. 8–7). Less than half of the femoral head or the whole head may be involved.

Clinically, the hip is stiff and painful and the patient may limp and complain of knee pain. The goal of treatment is to ensure that the femoral head develops normally and assumes its normal round shape.[7] If half the femoral head is involved, the treatment consists of rest. If the whole head is involved, the patient wears a brace or cast that effectively contains the head in the acetabulum while healing takes place. In severe cases of Perthes disease, a varus or innominate osteotomy may be performed.[7]

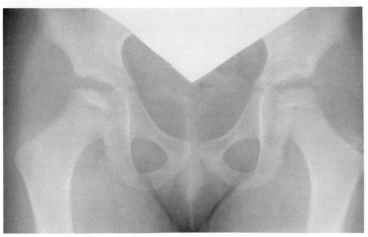

Figure 8–7
Early avascular necrosis of the right femoral epiphysis.

Initial radiographs include anteroposterior and frog-leg lateral views of both hips to compare the size of the affected epiphysis with the healthy side (Fig. 8–8). The frog-leg lateral view is often the more informative, as the resorption process tends to take place anterolaterally.[8] In the earlier phases of Perthes disease, a ^{99m}Tc bone scan may show a bone defect before it is visible on radiographs. The bone scan will show a decrease or lack of uptake of the radionuclide at the site of the avascular necrosis (Fig. 8–9).

Positive-contrast hip arthrography may be performed to evaluate the outline of the cartilaginous femoral head. However, ultrasonography and magnetic resonance imaging (both are noninvasive and nonionizing radiation modalities) are now used at many facilities to check for joint fluid, marrow edema, and the degree of necrosis.

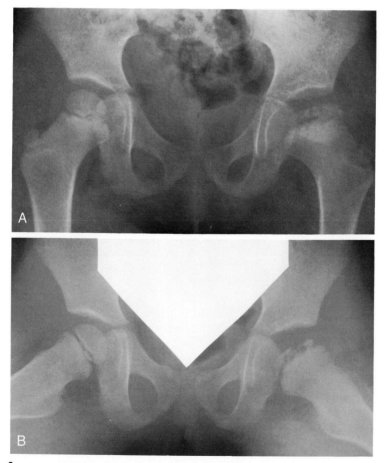

Figure 8–8

A, Anteroposterior and **B**, frog-leg lateral views showing flattening of the femoral epiphysis and metaphysis, with fragmentation of the epiphyseal ossification center on the left. Some resorption of bony fragments is consistent with healing in Legg-Calvé-Perthes disease.

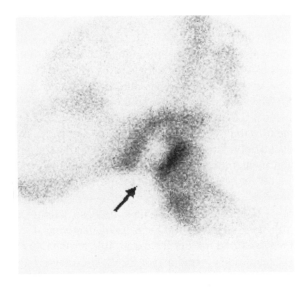

Figure 8-9
Radionuclide study showing a
decrease in uptake in the area of
avascular necrosis (*arrow*).

> **Routine Projections:** Anteroposterior and frog-leg lateral. Use gonadal shielding without obscuring the hip joints.

SLIPPED CAPITAL FEMORAL EPIPHYSIS

An SCFE is a Salter-Harris type I fracture of the growth plate of the proximal femur during the period of accelerated growth that takes place at puberty.[4] The incidence varies according to the child's race, sex, and geographic location.[9] The risk is slightly greater for Black males and is more common in the eastern than southwestern United States.[9] Incidence is greater in males between ages 12 and 15 years and in females between ages 10 and 13 years.[4] The male-female ratio is 3 : 1, and peak incidence occurs at puberty. Patients are generally obese and slightly tall for their age, and skeletal maturation is delayed.[4]

Although the reason for SCFE is obscure, increased body weight and delayed skeletal maturation are considered to contribute to a decrease in strength of the growth plate and an increase in the amount of shearing stress to which the growth plate is subjected.[4] Also, more than half of the patients have sustained a trauma before the diagnosis of SCFE.[4]

The slip may be gradual or sudden; severity is graded I, II, and III. Grade I is a minimal slip, grade II is a marked slip without avascular necrosis, and grade III is a marked slip with avascular necrosis.[4] In 25% to 30% of cases, both hips are involved; this occurs more frequently in females.[4] The left hip is affected more than the right in males.[8]

Clinical symptoms of a gradual slip are a limp, hip pain, and/or referred knee pain. In an acute slip, there is a sudden onset of severe pain in the hip, motion is restricted, and the patient is unable to bear weight. While the patient is recumbent, the affected hip and leg assume a laterally rotated position. An acute slip occurs in two forms: acute traumatic after an injury, and acute on chronic when the patient suddenly experiences severe pain after months or weeks of pain in the hip or thigh.[9]

Movement is extremely painful, and these patients must be handled gently and very carefully. The condition is a surgical emergency, and the patient may be a candidate for reduction and traction followed by pin fixation or may require an immediate hip-pinning procedure. Treatment involves stabilizing the hip to prevent further slippage of the epiphysis.[7]

An SCFE is sometimes difficult to see on an anteroposterior radiograph, and the frog-leg lateral or true lateral view is critical in making an accurate diagnosis. A suspected SCFE will be seen as a metaphyseal-epiphyseal step because of the displacement of the epiphysis, with offset of the margins of the epiphysis and the metaphysis visible on the frog-leg lateral view[8] (Fig. 8–10). Posterior displacement occurs in 99% and medial displacement in 75% of cases.[8]

If the slip is acute and the hip is too painful to move, the horizontal ray lateral position avoids the stress of the frog-leg lateral position.[3] Unfortunately, a true lateral projection is difficult to obtain with these patients as the hip is too painful to move, and if they are overweight there is a large amount of scatter. When radiographing an adult for a fractured neck of the femur, it is reasonably easy to see the neck on a true lateral radiograph. To demonstrate SCFE, the radiographer must try to show the complete head of the femur and the acetabulum on the lateral view, a challenge with an obese patient. A 400-speed screen/film combination, a high-ratio grid, precise centering, and collimation are required to obtain good results.

Treatment of young patients involves stabilization of the slip to prevent further displacement until after the physis closes.[3] If blood supply to the femoral head is compromised, avascular necrosis and, later in life, osteoarthritis may occur.[3] SCFE is treated as an emergency. The patient is admitted and the hip put in traction, followed by in situ fixation. Fixation of the femoral epiphysis to the metaphysis and femoral neck by single or multiple pins is performed in the operating room.

The hip-pinning procedure should be performed under fluoroscopy, with a mobile image intensifier that can easily be positioned for both anteroposterior and lateral radiographs. Pulsed imaging—not continual fluoroscopy—is used to minimize radiation dose. The image intensifier should be controlled by a radiographer who is responsible for positioning, keeping track of the number of pulses, and recording the pulses on the patient requisition form.

A guide wire is inserted into the upper femur, the femoral neck, and then the femoral head and the epiphyseal plate. The guide wire enables the surgeon to determine the correct pin or screw placement. Either a fixation pin is placed alongside the guide wire or a cannulated screw is placed over it (Fig. 8–11). The guide wire is then

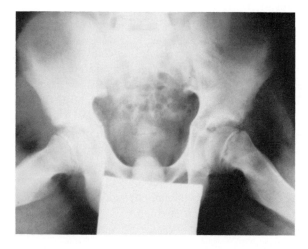

Figure 8–10

Frog-leg lateral view of both hips, showing a slipped capital femoral epiphysis on the left.

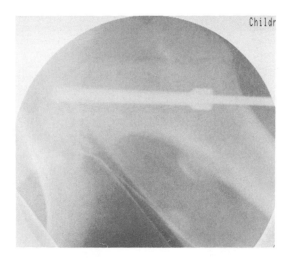

Figure 8-11

Image taken during fluoroscopic procedure in the operating room, showing the position of the cannulated screw over the guide wire.

withdrawn. It is important to ensure that the screw does not penetrate the hip joint. The device is designed for easy removal after the epiphysis has closed.

One screw or pin is used on most patients, but this depends on the severity of the slip and the size or weight of the patient (Fig. 8-12). The femoral epiphyseal plate closes in 4 to 6 months.

FRACTURES

Fractures of the hip and pelvis are common in elderly people but uncommon in children.[1] Osteoporotic bone is fragile, while the growing bone of children is more resilient. Most pelvic fractures in children are simple and undisplaced and are usually of the pubic bones as the result of a motor vehicle or car/pedestrian accident. The bladder and lower urinary tract are also vulnerable to injury when the pubic bone is fractured.[1]

Common injuries of the pelvis include avulsion fractures, which occur in adolescents. Avulsion fractures, which are sports related, result from a sudden pull on a

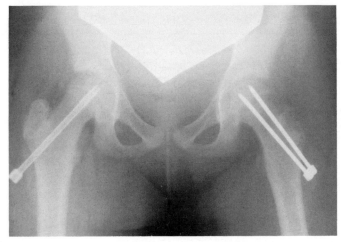

Figure 8-12

Anteroposterior view of both hips, showing one cannulated screw in the right hip and two fixation pins in the left hip.

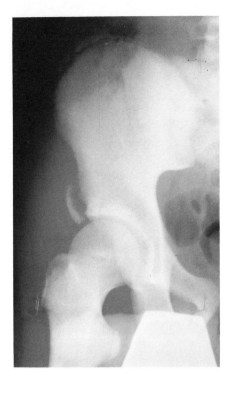

Figure 8–13

Avulsion fracture of the right anterior superior iliac spine incurred by a 13-year-old male performing a high jump.

muscle during vigorous athletic activity, detaching the apophysis from its normal position.[8] The apophyses are growth centers of bone like the epiphyses, but they do not contribute to growth in the length of a bone. Apophyses serve as muscle attachments, of which the four most common sites in the pelvis are the ASIS, the anterior inferior iliac spine, (AIIS), the ischial tuberosity, and the iliac crest[1] (Fig. 8–13).

Sprinters, hurdlers, football players, and ballet dancers are candidates for avulsion fractures.[8] After an apophysis is detached, a large amount of callus may form around the site, mimicking a malignant bone tumor.[8] A standard anteroposterior projection of the pelvis is usually all that is required, and it is one of the few instances in which gonadal shielding should *not* be used.

Routine Projection: Anteroposterior, whole pelvis without gonadal shielding.

REFERENCES

1. Houston, C.S., Pelvis and hips, in Pediatric Skeletal Radiology, pp. 310–346, M.H. Reed, Ed., Williams & Wilkins, Baltimore, 1992
2. Risser, J.G., The iliac apophysis: An invaluable sign in the management of scoliosis, Clinical Orthopedics, 11:111–119, 1958
3. Ozonoff, M.B., Pediatric Orthopedic Radiology, 2nd ed., W.B. Saunders Company, Philadelphia, 1992
4. Sty, J.R., Wells, R.G., Starshak, R.J., et al., Diagnostic Imaging of Infants and Children, Vol. 3, Aspen Publishers, Gaithersburg, 1992
5. Silverman, F.N., Kuhn, J.P., Caffey's Pediatric X-ray Diagnosis. An Integrated Approach, Vol. I, 9th ed., C.V. Mosby Company, St. Louis, 1993
6. Andrén, L., von Rosen, S., The diagnosis of the hip in newborns and the primary results of immediate treatment, Acta Radiologica, 49:89–95, 1958
7. Wenger, D.R., and Rang, M., The Art and Practice of Children's Orthopedics, Raven Press, New York, 1993
8. Oestreich, A.E., Skeletal system, in Practical Pediatric Imaging: Diagnostic Radiology of Infants and Children, 2nd ed., pp. 263–415, D.R. Kirks, Ed., Little, Brown & Company, Boston, 1991
9. Tachdjian, M.O., Pediatric Orthopedics, 2nd ed., W.B. Saunders Company, Philadelphia, 1990

The Skull

DEVELOPMENT

Skull, *cranium*, and *calvaria* are terms used to describe the skull. Although skull and cranium are used interchangeably, the literature suggests that skull includes the head, face, and mandible; cranium excludes the mandible; and calvaria excludes the facial bones.[1] The calvaria consists of eight bones: the frontal, ethmoid, sphenoid, occipital, and the paired parietal and temporal bones. The 14 facial bones are the nasal, lacrimal, maxillary, zygomatic, palatine, inferior nasal concha, ethmoid, and vomer bones.

The bones of the skull develop from mesenchyma around the developing brain.[2] The skull consists of the neurocranium (the protective bony case of the brain) and the viscerocranium (which forms the upper and lower jaws). Ossification within the membranous neurocranium during fetal life forms the bones of the calvaria.[2]

The bones of the calvaria are flat and thin and are separated by tough, fibrous connective tissue along the sagittal, coronal, lamboid, metopic, and squamosal sutures. These loose, fibrous connections enable the calvaria to change shape during birth. As the fetus passes through the birth canal, the frontal bone becomes flat, the occiput is drawn out, and one parietal bone overrides the other. Soon after birth the skull assumes its normal, much rounder shape.

Expansions of fibrous tissue along the sutures are called fontanelles, six of which are present at birth. The largest, the bregma, is at the junction of the metopic, coronal, and sagittal sutures. It is diamond shaped and overlies the superior sagittal dural venous sinus. Arterial pumping of blood into the brain causes the bregma to pulsate. The posterior fontanelle, the lambda, is at the junction of the lambdoid and sagittal sutures. The lambda closes by about 3 months and the bregma between 6 and 20 months of age.[2]

As the skull grows, the suture lines gradually become serrated and interdigitate, eventually closing in adolescence or adulthood. Prenatal closure of a suture or sutures, a condition called craniosynostosis, results in an abnormally shaped head.[2] The growth of the calvaria is perpendicular to the suture lines; the type of deformity depends on which of the sutures is synostotic. The most common prenatal fusion (60% of all cases) is sagittal synostosis; this condition results in elongation of the skull.[2] If the coronal suture closes early, the head will be wide from side to side but shallow from front to back. Skull asymmetry results when a suture closes unilaterally.

The bones of a newborn skull are very thin. It is difficult to see suture lines on a radiograph, as the membranous bone fades into the fibrous tissue. Unlike the bony cranium in the adult, the calvaria of the neonate appears almost featureless, although crescent-shaped lines from folds of loose scalp tissue are sometimes seen on skull radiographs (Fig. 9–1). Hair braids, dirt, and electroencephalography paste are also more likely to show up as artifacts on younger children, sometimes mimicking calcifications within the brain.

The head of a neonate is large in proportion to the rest of the body, and the facial area is small compared with the calvaria. The ratio on a lateral skull radiograph of the size of the facial bones to the cranial vault is 4:1 in a newborn compared with 1.5:1 in an adult[1] (Fig. 9–2). This is because of the small jaws, absence of teeth, small nasal cavity, and rudimentary characteristics of the paranasal sinuses. Although the skull as a whole grows relatively less than do other parts of the skeleton, it is a dynamic, changing structure in a child. The greatest increase occurs in the first 2 years of life, which is also the time of the most rapid growth of the brain.

As the skull develops, developmental variations may occur, many of which are insignificant. One example is wormian bones, named after Worm, the Danish anatomist. These are small accessory bones that develop in sutures, particularly in the

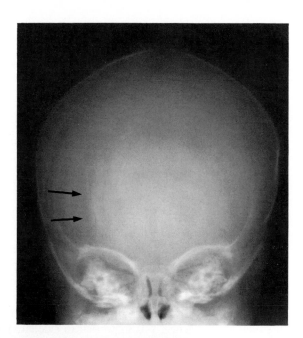

Figure 9–1

Anteroposterior view of the skull of a newborn showing crescent-shaped artifacts from folds of scalp tissue (*arrows*).

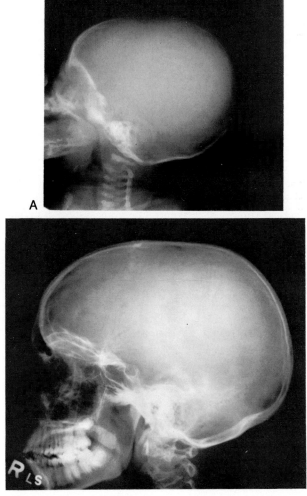

Figure 9–2

Comparison of the relative size of the facial bones and calvaria in **A**, a newborn skull and **B**, an adult skull.

lambdoid suture.[3] They are usually considered normal variants, although multiple wormian bones are found in children with developmental disorders such as cretinism and osteogenesis imperfecta.

The vascular and convolutional markings seen on the inner surface of the calvaria in adults are not present in the newborn but develop as the skull and brain develop.[4] They reflect normal brain development and pattern the surface of the cerebrum and cerebellum. Brain growth is 60% complete by 12 months of age, 80% complete by 3 years, and 95% complete by 8 years.[4]

RADIOGRAPHIC TECHNIQUE

Pediatric skull radiography has always been an art rather than an exact science. The head is a growing, constantly changing structure in young children, so it is difficult to be specific as to the exact angle and position for the various projections. A radiographer experienced in pediatric skull radiography has always been the key to good, consistent diagnostic radiographs, but currently there are fewer radiographers with that type of experience. It is important to evaluate facial characteristics and to realize that less tube and skull angulation is needed in younger children than in adolescents or adults.

Significantly fewer conventional radiographs of the skull are taken today, as a variety of noninvasive imaging modalities are available for imaging the skull and central nervous system. Computed tomography (CT), magnetic resonance imaging (MRI), and ultrasonography have replaced most earlier invasive imaging procedures of the brain, notably pneumoencephalography and air ventriculography.

Ultrasonography is particularly useful for evaluating the brain of the newborn through the anterior fontanelle.[5] Neonates born prematurely are at risk for intracranial hemorrhage, specifically, germinal matrix hemorrhage and intraventricular hemorrhage. Mobile real-time ultrasonography is usually the preferred examination in the neonatal intensive care unit, because it is easier to move an ultrasound machine than a baby with all the life support systems.[5]

Pediatric neuroradiology, a subspecialty of radiology, covers a vast array of diseases and conditions. Tumors of the central nervous system are common in childhood, after leukemia the second most common pediatric malignant disease.[4] Because tumors, congenital malformations, and infections are mainly evaluated by CT and MRI, this chapter is limited to the more common pediatric conditions that are still evaluated by conventional skull radiography.

> **Technical Considerations:** The three standard skull projections can be performed on a regular x-ray table. Preferably, a skull unit or an upright stand should be available for erect views of the paranasal sinuses. An extension or a sinus cone helps reduce scatter but does not preclude the use of tight collimation. A 400-speed screen/film system gives satisfactory resolution for the lowest patient radiation dose.

SKULL TRAUMA

At Children's Hospital, after cervical spine films are taken, patients with head trauma and other patients when indicated are usually transported directly from the emergency room to the CT scanner. Although the value of plain radiographs for evaluating skull injuries has been debated for a number of years,[4,6,7] skull radiographs are still requested by many physicians in hospitals without immediate access to CT.

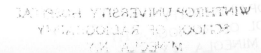

Studies show that the presence of a calvarial fracture does not always indicate significant intracranial injury, and the absence of a skull fracture does not rule out a serious neurologic finding. Patton[8] says that skull radiographs are greatly overused in the evaluation of children with head trauma. Conventional skull radiography does not alter the clinical management of these patients, except for those with a depressed or compound fracture.[6]

Head trauma is a leading cause of morbidity and death in children.[2,9] In the United States, head injuries cause more deaths in children between the ages of 1 and 19 years than all other diseases combined.[10] Motor vehicle accidents are the most common cause, followed by pedestrian accidents, particularly between the ages of 5 and 9 years.

Infants are more prone to head injuries than older children, as their brains have less protection. There is less myelination, and the fontanelles are still open. An infant's neck is flexible and pliable, so the head is shaken around more easily. Infant car seats are often incorrectly placed, facing forward instead of backward, leading to an increased risk of subdural hematoma and whiplash if a car is involved in a collision.

Children who fall from heights are more likely than adults to suffer from head injuries. The theory is that because their heads are relatively larger than their torsos, their center of gravity is higher, and they tend to fall head first.[9]

In children under age 5, a short fall from a couch or bed rarely results in significant intracranial injury.[11] Fractures and life-threatening intracranial injuries in a child are more often consistent with having been shaken or battered, rather than having fallen from a bed. Ninety-five percent of serious head injuries in children under age 5 years are the result of child abuse and are a major social issue in many industrialized countries.[9,11]

Anteroposterior and lateral skull radiographs are an essential part of a skeletal survey in cases of suspected child abuse. For example, a small linear fracture seen in these radiographs may be an important indication of abuse and may warrant placing a child under the protection of the Department of Social Services. One important point: when child abuse is suspected, the radiographer should not tell the parent or guardian accompanying the child the reason for a skeletal survey. The child may have been brought to the emergency room for a relatively minor injury, and the physician or nurse examining the child may see or suspect other unexplained trauma. If the person or persons accompanying the child are responsible for the abuse and become aware they are under suspicion, they are apt to leave the hospital abruptly.

For the general survey of the skull, three projections are usually sufficient: anteroposterior, anteroposterior axial (Townes), and lateral.

RADIOGRAPHIC POSITIONING

Most radiographers find positioning and immobilizing infants and toddlers for skull radiographs challenging, probably more so since the advent of CT. Fewer plain radiographs are taken, which has decreased the opportunity to use skull-positioning skills on a regular basis.

Immobilization and positioning is easier with the child supine, because young children enjoy watching the activity around them. Trying to obtain a straight, unrotated view of the skull in a posteroanterior position is almost impossible. Toddlers and preschoolers also find it less frightening to lie on their backs rather than have their noses pressed against the x-ray table.

Objections to the anteroposterior projection are based on the long-standing recommended practice of positioning a patient facing away from the x-ray tube to protect the lens of the eye from the entrance radiation exposure. Although both the patient position and the radiation dose are important technical considerations, patient comfort and the avoidance of a repeat radiograph are of equal importance. When assessing anteroposterior versus posteroanterior in this instance, the entrance exposure for an anteroposterior skull radiograph is low and the dose negligible, particularly in comparison to the estimated 4 rad for a standard head CT scan. According to the dose tables in Chapter 15, the exposure for an anteroposterior or a posteroanterior skull radiograph, using a 400-speed screen/film combination, depending on age, is between 16 and 65 mrad.

Infants and toddlers may be immobilized by the mummy-wrapping technique described in Chapter 10. A pacifier helps calm a baby or small infant. A preschool or school-age child may be comforted by holding a favorite toy or blanket during the procedure. Unless state law specifically forbids it, a parent should stay in the room and hold the child's hand. Always try to talk a child through the procedure before resorting to restraints—depending on the age group, being restrained may only add to the fears of an already frightened child.

Routine Projections: For patients from newborn to 8 years of age: anteroposterior, anteroposterior axial (Townes), and lateral.

Anteroposterior (Fig. 9–3)

The patient is supine, with the head positioned so that the midsagittal plane and the orbitomeatal line are perpendicular to the table. The central ray is perpendicular to the glabella. Because the frontal sinuses are small and there is little aeration, the

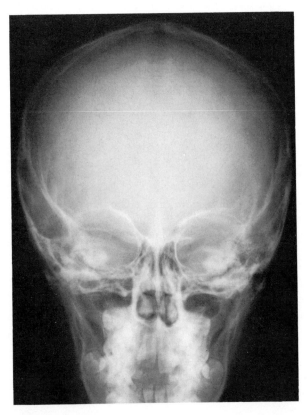

Figure 9–3

Anteroposterior view of the skull of an 8-year-old child.

view of the parietal and frontal bones on the radiograph is unobstructed. The petrous ridges are seen through the orbits. A 5- to 15-degree caudad angulation may be needed on an older child, depending on the degree of facial development.

Anteroposterior Axial (Townes) (Fig. 9–4)

The patient is positioned the same as for the anteroposterior projection. The central ray is angled at 20 to 25 degrees caudad and exits at the level of the foramen magnum. Because children are usually much more flexible than adults, there is a tendency for the neck to be flexed too much, or for the caudal angulation to be too great. On the resultant radiograph, the posterior arch of the atlas is seen high in the foramen magnum, with foreshortening of the occipital bone. Remember, the facial bones are small compared with the calvaria in this age group, so less caudal angulation is required than for the adult skull.

Lateral (Fig. 9–5)

If there is neck trauma, the lateral projection is taken with a cross-table horizontal x-ray beam. As with adults, this same lateral projection is also routine for skull trauma once the sphenoidal air sinus is radiologically visible. A fluid level in the sinus may be the only radiologic indication of a fracture through the base of the skull.

Depending on the injury and the age of the child, the lateral projection can be taken with the head turned to one side. Because the cranium is relatively large compared with the mandible and thorax, a foam pad placed under the shoulders and neck, as well as under the jaw, with the contralateral shoulder slightly raised, helps to maintain the head in a true lateral position. The head should be adjusted until the median sagittal plane is parallel and the interpupillary line is perpendicular to the

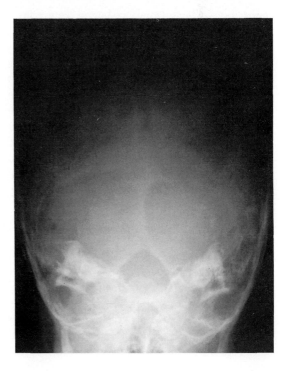

Figure 9–4
Anteroposterior axial view of the skull of an 8-year-old child.

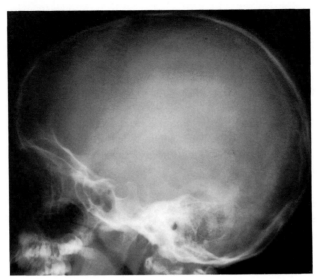

Figure 9–5
Lateral view of the skull of an 8-year-old child.

table. The central ray is perpendicular and centered midway between the glabella and the occiput. The centering point should be adjusted for a head that is enlarged, as in hydrocephalus, or asymmetrical, as in craniosynostosis.

Children over age 8 may be positioned as adults, although this depends on the degree of facial development, temperament, and type of trauma or condition.

HYDROCEPHALUS

Cerebrospinal fluid (CSF) is secreted by the choroid plexus, mainly in the lateral ventricles. It flows from the lateral ventricles into the third ventricle through the foramen of Monro and from the third into the fourth ventricle via the aqueduct of Sylvius. It passes from the fourth ventricle into the subarachnoid spaces through the midline foramen of Magendie and the paired lateral foramina of Luschka. CSF is eventually absorbed into the venous circulation through the arachnoid villi.

The flow of CSF, sometimes considered the third circulation, provides a highly specialized environment for the brain and spinal cord. Hydrocephalus is a pathologic condition with many variations and is characterized by an increased amount of CSF, with ventricular enlargement and an increase in CSF pressure.

Hydrocephalus may be classified as noncommunicating or communicating. Noncommunicating hydrocephalus results from an obstruction proximal to the outlet of the fourth ventricle.[12] It may be due to a congenital abnormality (such as aqueductus stenosis), a tumor, or an inflammatory condition. There is no blockage with communicating hydrocephalus, but the amount of CSF absorbed is less than that produced. Both conditions in young children result in enlarged ventricles, increased intracranial pressure, and, depending on age, widened sutures.[12]

Imaging techniques include CT and MRI, but conventional radiographs are useful in evaluating shunts. A shunting procedure may be performed to bypass the obstruction to the flow of CSF. A shunt assists in decreasing intracranial pressure to safe—if not normal—values and in increasing the volume of brain tissue.[12]

Most shunting systems are valve regulated. The differential pressure across the valve regulates the rate of flow to prevent overdrainage and ventricular collapse.[10] The procedure consists of placing one end of a plastic tube within a lateral ventricle, anterior to the foramen of Monro and proximal to the site of the obstruction. The tubing is passed in a subcutaneous tunnel down the side of the neck and into the right atrium or peritoneal cavity.[12] The latter route is more commonly used as the tubing can be coiled into the peritoneal cavity, uncoiling as the child grows (Fig. 9–6). This alleviates the number of times a shunt has to be revised during childhood.

There is always a risk of infection with a shunt, whether it is ventricle to peritoneum (V-P) or ventricle to atrium (V-A).[12] A distal infection in a V-P shunt is less of a risk than in the V-A shunt, which can be life threatening. Other complications include broken tubing, disconnection, obstruction, hematoma, and thromboembolism.[12] CT and MRI are used to evaluate ventricular size, but plain radiographs satisfactorily evaluate the course and position of the shunt tubing.

To properly evaluate a shunt, the complete length of the tubing must be visible on both frontal and lateral radiographs. Recumbent anteroposterior and lateral projections of the skull, chest, and abdomen are necessary to cover the entire length of a V-P shunt (Fig. 9–7). On the lateral projections (to visualize the shunt, which is percutaneous), the neck, chest, and abdomen should be slightly underexposed. Recumbent anteroposterior and lateral projections of the skull and neck and of the chest and abdomen provide satisfactory coverage in a younger child. Older children require separate radiographs of the chest and abdomen.

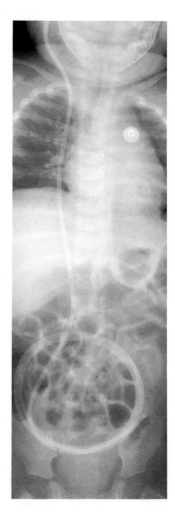

Figure 9–6

Coiled tubing in the lower abdomen in a ventricle-peritoneum shunt in a 1-year-old child.

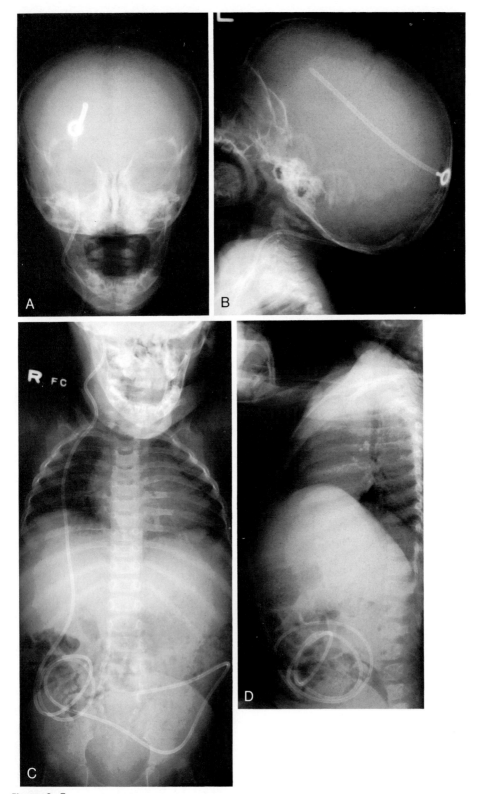

Figure 9–7
Radiographs of the skull, chest, and abdomen, showing intact tubing in a ventricle-peritoneum shunt in a 4-month-old with myelodysplasia. **A,** Anteroposterior view of skull. **B,** Lateral view of skull. **C,** Anteroposterior view of chest and abdomen. **D,** Lateral view of chest and abdomen. Note the sacral deformity and bilateral hip dysplasia.

To evaluate a V-A shunt, anteroposterior and lateral projections of the skull, and an anteroposterior and anteroposterior oblique projection of the chest, should be taken. In this instance, the right posterior oblique position demonstrates the position of the tubing in the right atrium better than does the lateral position.

Routine Projections: V-P shunt: Recumbent anteroposterior and lateral views of the skull, neck, chest, and abdomen. V-A shunt: Recumbent anteroposterior, and lateral views of the skull, recumbent anteroposterior, and recumbent position views of the chest.

PARANASAL SINUSES

The paranasal sinuses are paired frontal, ethmoid, sphenoid, and maxillary cells filled with air that develop as outpouchings of the nasal mucous membrane. All the sinuses communicate with the nasal cavity. The size and extent of aeration vary considerably at different ages and in different individuals.

The maxillary sinuses are present at birth but are not radiographically visible until 2 to 3 months of age.[4] The ethmoid sinuses parallel the growth of the maxillary sinuses but are smaller and not radiographically visible until 3 to 6 months. Both reach adult size at about 10 to 12 years. The sphenoid sinuses may be aerated as early as 1 to 2 years but do not reach adult size until 14 years. The frontal sinuses begin development as early as 1 year but are not radiologically visible until 8 to 10 years.[4] Radiologic interpretation is more difficult with children than adults as these sinuses are smaller and less distinct from the surrounding structures.[4]

Children who are old enough to sit or stand should be radiographed upright, facing a skull table or an upright stand containing a stationary or moving grid. Many departments no longer have specialized skull units as there is less need for complex skull examinations. At Children's Hospital we no longer need a specialized skull unit; we use a trauma unit with interchangeable cassette trays. It is similar to a skull unit in that the tube and stand move as a unit, rather like a mobile C-arm. It does not have the versatility of a skull unit but works well for erect views of the paranasal sinuses. This trauma unit is not a cheap substitute, but it costs much less than a custom-designed unit for this particular examination for pediatric patients.

RADIOGRAPHIC POSITIONING

Routine Projections: Over age 3: Posteroanterior, parietoacanthial, and lateral.

Posteroanterior (Fig. 9–8)

The patient stands or sits facing the upright stand with forehead and nose on the stand. The midsagittal plane and orbitomeatal line are at right angles to the plane of the film. A straight tube is used in a younger child and is centered to the nasion. Progressively, a caudal angulation of 5 to 15 degrees is used, depending on the age of the child. This view shows the frontal and anterior ethmoid sinuses.

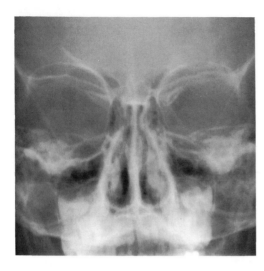

Figure 9–8

Posteroanterior view showing developing ethmoid and frontal sinuses in a 6-year-old child.

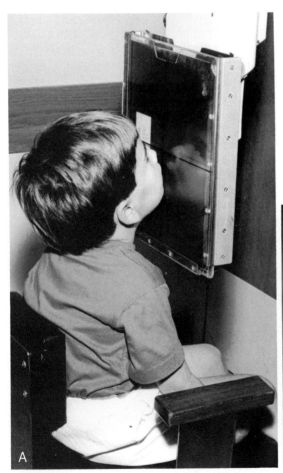

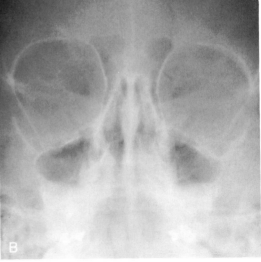

Figure 9–9

A, A 6-year-old boy in position for a parietoacanthial projection of the sinuses. *B*, Parieto-acanthial view, showing well-aerated maxillary antra.

Parietoacanthial (Waters Method) (Fig. 9–9)

The patient stands or sits facing the upright stand with the neck extended and the chin on the stand. The major problem in positioning children for this view is that the neck is frequently overextended so that the maxillary antra are foreshortened. This foreshortening results in a less than optimal study and a possible error in diagnosis. The orbitomeatal line should be adjusted, depending on age and facial development, at an angle between 20 and 35 degrees to the plane of the film, rather than the 37 degrees recommended for adults.

It is difficult to be specific because of differences in growth and facial contours, but it helps to have a mental image of the relationship of the petrous pyramids to the maxillae while positioning the patient's head. The objective is to ensure that the petrous pyramids do not overlap the floor of the antra, as this view gives the most information on the condition of the maxillary sinuses. The central ray is at right angles to the film at the level of the acanthion.

Lateral (Fig. 9–10)

This projection shows the superimposed frontal, ethmoid, and maxillary sinuses and sphenoids, depending on development and aeration. When adults are radiographed, the head is usually turned to one side for the lateral projection, giving an

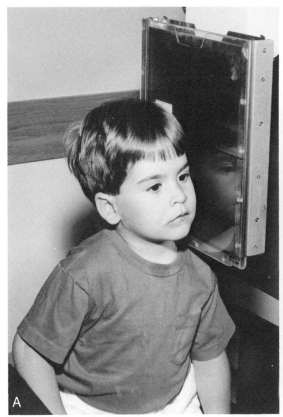
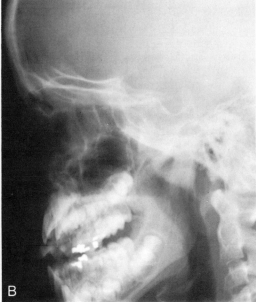

Figure 9–10
A, A 6-year-old boy in position for a true lateral projection of the sinuses. **B**, Lateral view, showing superimposition of the frontal, ethmoid, and maxillary sinuses and the upper airway. Aeration of the sphenoidal sinuses is beginning.

oblique view of the upper airway. With children, however, it is important to include the entire upper airway, so the head and neck should be in a true lateral position. Frequently both the sinuses and the upper respiratory tract are infected, as they are anatomically in close proximity. The adenoids also need to be evaluated in children. The patient is positioned standing or sitting, with the head and neck in true lateral position, shoulders depressed, and chin slightly extended. If the patient is able to cooperate, this projection can be done, like the others, at an upright stand.

Another method is to position the patient the same way as for a lateral view of the neck. Include the sinuses and airway and use a 72-inch SID to minimize magnification. A grid is not necessary for younger children. The central ray is at right angles and centered to the center of the film, approximately 1 inch posterior and 1 inch below the outer canthus of the eye, remote from the film. For children over 8 years of age, separate radiographs of the airway and lateral sinuses may be required.

Routine Projections: Patients 1 to 3 years of age: Anteroposterior, reverse Waters method, and lateral.

It is much easier to position and immobilize children in this age group lying down, although some 3-year-olds may be able to maintain the correct position without motion when standing or sitting.

Anteroposterior (Fig. 9–11)

The patient is supine, as for an anteroposterior skull projection, with the central ray perpendicular to the nasion.

Reverse Waters Method (Fig. 9–12)

The patient is supine, with the chin elevated until the orbitomeatal line forms a 15- to 20-degree angle with the table and the central ray is perpendicular to the acanthion.

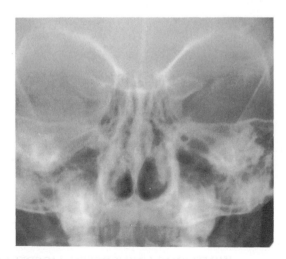

Figure 9–11

Supine, anteroposterior view, showing ethmoid sinuses in a 3-year-old child. The frontal sinuses are not yet aerated.

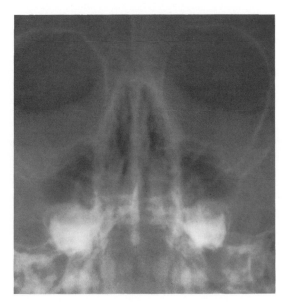

Figure 9–12

Supine, anteroposterior view (reverse Waters method), showing aerated maxillary antra in a 3-year-old child. Note the tooth buds at the base of the antra.

Lateral

The patient may be sitting or supine. If the child is sitting, the positioning and centering is the same as for an older child. If the child is supine, elevate the head and neck on a radiolucent foam block and place a cassette at the side of the head to include the face and upper airway in the radiograph. The horizontal beam is centered to the center of the film.

REFERENCES

1. Shapiro, R., Radiology of the Normal Skull, 1981 Yearbook, Medical Publishers, Chicago, 1981
2. Sty, J.R., Wells, R.G., Starshak, R.G., et al., Diagnostic Imaging of Infants and Children, Vol. 2, Aspen Publishers, Gaithersburg, MD, 1992
3. Ramsey, R.G., Neuroradiology, W.B. Saunders, Philadelphia, 1987
4. Ball, W.S., and Prenger, E.C., Skull and contents, in Practical Pediatric Imaging: Diagnostic Radiology of Infants and Children, 2nd ed., pp. 57–91, D.R. Kirks, Ed., Little, Brown & Company, Boston, 1991
5. Teele, R.L., and Share, J.C., Ultrasonography of Infants and Children, W.B. Saunders Company, Philadelphia, 1991
6. Harwood-Nash, D.C., Hendrick, E.B., and Hudson, A.R., The significance of skull fractures in children, Radiology, 101:151–155, 1971
7. Leonidas, J.C., Windsor, T., Binkiewicz, A., et al., Mild head trauma in children: When is a roentgenogram necessary?, Pediatrics, 69(2):139–143, 1982
8. Patton, A., Skull, in Pediatric Skeletal Radiology, pp. 171–189, M.H. Reed, Ed., Williams & Wilkins, Baltimore, 1982
9. Reed, M.H., Trauma in Pediatric Skeletal Radiology, pp. 108–125, M.H. Reed, Ed., Williams & Wilkins, Baltimore, 1982
10. Division of Injury Control, Center for Environmental Health and Injury Control, Centers for Disease Control. Childhood Injuries in the United States, American Journal of Diseases of Children, 144:627–646, 1990
11. Billmire, M.E., and Myers, P.A., Serious head injury in infants: Accident or abuse?, Pediatrics, 75(2):340–342, 1985
12. McLaurin, R.L., Pediatric Neurosurgery, 2nd ed., W.B. Saunders, Philadelphia, 1989

Immobilization

Linda Poznauskis

POSITIONING DEVICES

One of the delightful aspects of working with children is their spontaneity and unpredictability. These characteristics make it extremely important to have and know how to properly use restraining and positioning devices.

As with adults, positioning devices help maintain a desired position and ensure the safety of the patient. A restraining device works best when there is no space between the patient and the device. A sponge or towel may be needed to make the restraining device fit snugly, effectively helping to maintain the correct position. This is not only helpful with a very young or incapacitated child, but necessary, because most x-ray tables are equipped with a compression band designed for adults. The use of sandbags, towels, or radiolucent sponges to fill in spaces keeps the child safe and in position (Fig. 10–1).

Positioning devices also have a calming effect. Babies, for instance, are used to being swaddled in blankets and clothing. Babies and small children who have been wrapped in sheets to restrain their movement may actually calm down because they feel safer swaddled than uncovered.

Children with a condition such as cerebral palsy, in which muscle contractions are likely to occur, should be immobilized so that their muscles are supported in their natural position. For example, to help a child with cerebral palsy who is unable to stand remain still for upright scoliosis spine radiographs, we lock a chair (ideally with removable sides and no back) in place. The patient sits on the chair, Velcro is strapped across the torso in several places, and blocks of wood are placed under the feet for support. The blocks under the feet will support the leg muscles in a natural position and prevent the leg-muscle contractions. The safer and more secure the patient feels, the better the opportunity for a satisfactory radiographic examination (Fig. 10–2).

It is important to remember that a child successfully immobilized requires fewer repeat radiographs, and thus minimal radiation exposure and less technologist time.

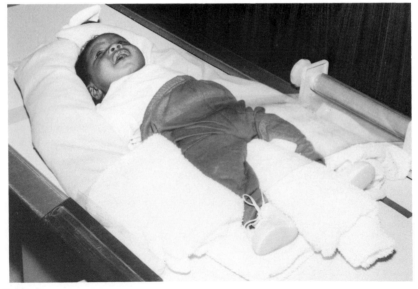

Figure 10–1
Padding the spaces makes the compression band fit snugly and keeps the child safe and in position.

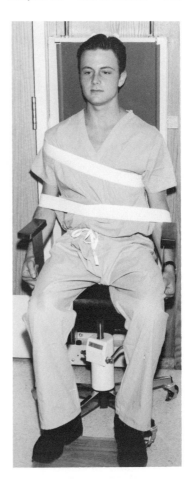

Figure 10-2
Wood blocks support the patient's feet and lower limbs, and Velcro straps support the torso for a sitting spine radiograph.

USING POSITIONING DEVICES CORRECTLY

Children present a particular challenge in that they are usually accompanied by parents who may be overwhelmed with concern because their child needs a radiographic examination. Parents can be an asset to the technologist, or they can create obstacles. It is essential that the procedure be explained to both the parents and the child. A parent can hold the child while you prepare the positioning devices. At the same time, explain to the parent what you are about to do. Demonstrate how you would like the parent to assist in positioning the child and why it is important to hold the child in a particular manner. We also give children the opportunity to position themselves whenever possible (Fig. 10-3). Most children are surprisingly willing if you give them the opportunity to feel comfortable and safe. Even a small child who needs a radiographic examination of the skull may be able to hold the radiolucent sponges as though they were earmuffs (with the gentle guidance of a parent) and thus be successfully immobilized.

A restraining device may be inappropriate at times. A child with an open wound or fracture, for instance, may not be a candidate for a restraining device. Babies 1 or 2 days after cardiac surgery should not be put in a Pigg-O-Stat, in which their arms need to be held straight above the head. It is important to visualize what impact a restraining device will have on the underlying anatomy before actually using a device.

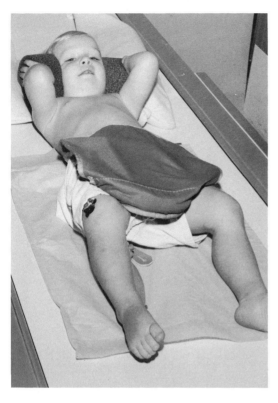

Figure 10-3
The child assists in positioning himself by holding the head sponges for an anteroposterior skull radiograph.

A child's first experience in the radiology department affects every successive visit. A child carelessly placed into a Pigg-O-Stat or other immobilization device without careful attention to his or her needs is likely to react negatively on a return visit. Patience and a little imagination can convince the child that sitting in a restraining device is not only nothing to be afraid of, but fun. Sometimes holding the child and coaxing him/her through the first examination means that no restraining device will be necessary on subsequent visits. Although coaxing is a preferred method, there may be legal constraints against holding patients in some states. In that case, restraining devices must be used.

MAKING THE MOST OF AVAILABLE MATERIALS

Tape, linens, disposables, radiolucent sponges, plexiglass, Velcro, and sandbags are inexpensive materials available in the radiology department (Fig. 10-4). Using them properly will save hours of wasted time and frustration.

TAPE

Tape is the easiest, least expensive item to use. It should not be difficult to remove, as some cloth tapes are, but should be strong enough to hold effectively. Paper tape breaks too easily. I recommend Johnson & Johnson[1] hypoallergenic tape, although it is expensive. When using tape for immobilization of the skull, a surgical pad (4 by 4 inch) over the forehead and under the tape prevents pain when the tape is removed. Make sure that the tape is attached to something secure on both ends.

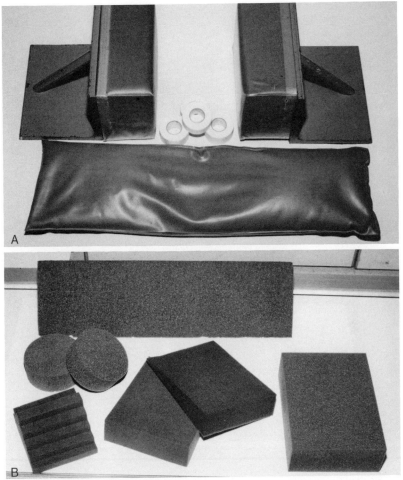

Figure 10–4
A, Hypoallergenic tape, sandbag, and head ends. *B*, Radiolucent sponges.

LINENS AND DISPOSABLES

Be sure there is an ample supply of sheets and towels. Sheets are particularly effective for total body immobilization. Place on the table a folded sheet that is about the height of the child. With the assistance of the parents or another technologist, place the child with the arms at the sides, and the head above and in the center of the sheet (Fig. 10–5A). Wrap the first side of the sheet so that it goes over the arm and under the torso (Fig. 10–5B). Repeat the wrap on the other side. Wrap another sheet totally around the child, or use a compression band or lead apron to finish immobilizing the child (Fig. 10–5C). Remember: If you don't take the time to properly immobilize the child before you begin the examination, you and the child will become frustrated. It is better to rewrap than to mistakenly believe that the child escaping from your first effort will stay still long enough to complete the examination.

For lateral skull radiographs on small babies, wrap a disposable paper underpad around the skull and then gently twist it anteriorly. Rotate the skull into the lateral position, maintaining the wrap, and use a sandbag or other heavy item (such as head ends) to hold the wrap down (Fig. 10–6). For an anteroposterior radiograph of the skull, the patient can be restrained by total body immobilization, as previously de-

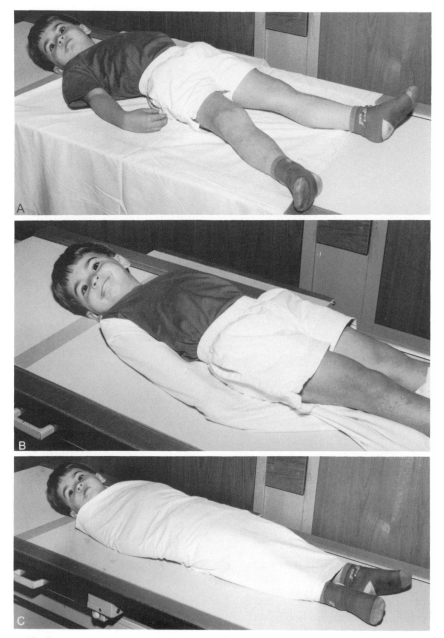

Figure 10–5
A, Starting a total body wrap with a folded sheet. **B,** The first side of the sheet is wrapped over the arm and under the torso. **C,** Another sheet is wrapped around the child, immobilizing his entire body.

scribed. Place a shallow triangular sponge under the head and immobilize with head ends or round sponges with sandbags on each side. Tape a surgical pad (4 by 4 inches) across the forehead.

RADIOLUCENT SPONGES

Stock your rooms with a minimal amount of inexpensive items, such as four flexible, washable, long sandbags (5 by 20 inches), radiolucent sponges of different

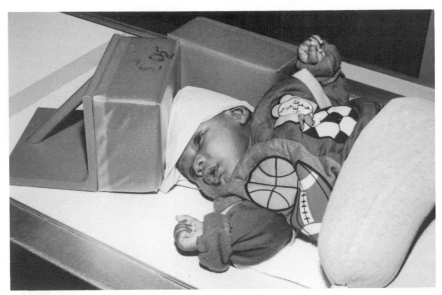

Figure 10–6
Immobilization with head ends, wrap, and sandbag for a lateral skull radiograph.

sizes, a pair of round sponges (3 inches thick, 7 inches in diameter), finger steps, a 45-degree long triangular sponge (7 by 7 by 14 inches), two angle sponges (12 to 14 degrees) that are about 7 inches wide, and a decubitus block (4 by 18 by 24 inches) (see Fig. 10–4B). Many companies now provide custom-made radiolucent sponges; Contour Fabricator is one example.[2]

PLEXIGLASS

Plexiglass strips, with the edges rounded, are useful. One company that makes these strips is Chamco, Inc.[3] The plexiglass strips are very effective for immobilizing hands and feet (Fig. 10–7).

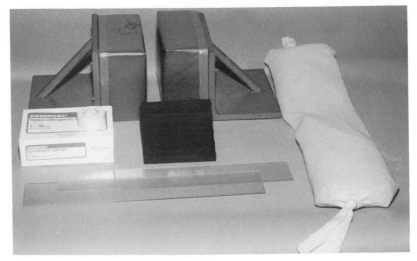

Figure 10–7
Head ends, plexiglass strips, tape, angled radiolucent sponge, and covered sandbag.

For an anteroposterior projection, the feet can be restrained by placing them flat on the cassette, with a strip of plexiglass across the feet secured by a sandbag on each end (Fig. 10–8). Be careful not to place the strip too high or too low on the feet. This creates extra space, making the restraint ineffective, and may allow the strips to cut into the foot. The lateral view can be done by placing a sandbag over the tibia and placing tape in several directions over the foot. Placing the foot in dorsiflexion using a head end will eliminate motion due to ankle flexion.

VELCRO

Velcro, another useful product, consists of hooks (the rough portion) and loops (the smooth portion). Both come with or without a glued back. Make sure the loop portion comes in contact with the patient and the hook portion is glued onto the inanimate object. Velcro, which comes by the piece or in strips, can be purchased from a radiology supply company[4] or in a fabric store. At Children's Hospital, we have placed Velcro on all of our chest stands to be used as a seat belt to restrain a fidgeting child (Fig. 10–9).

If an x-ray table does not have a compression band, Velcro can be used as a substitute. The hook portion should be glued onto the sides of the table and the loop portion used as the band. Velcro can be made sturdier by using two strips of hook parallel to each other on each end.

SANDBAGS

Sandbags are absolutely essential for taking chest radiographs of a baby, and the more sandbags used, the better. They are heavy and should be placed with the volume

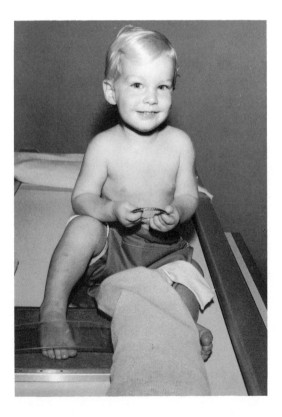

Figure 10–8

The patient's right foot is immobilized with a plexiglass strip held in place with sandbags for an anteroposterior radiograph.

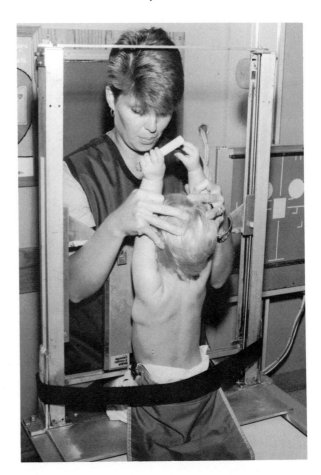

Figure 10–9

A Velcro strap restrains a seated child for a posteroanterior radiograph of the chest.

of sand on each side of the part to be immobilized — do not put the bulk of sand on the body.

When taking chest radiographs, place the infant in such a way that the head rests comfortably on the cassette. Do not let the baby's head rest on the edge of the cassette; this is painful and makes the baby uncomfortable. A cassette one size larger than usual is preferred. Abduct the arms and immobilize each with a sandbag (Fig. 10–10). If you abduct the arms enough, you will be able to use the ends of each sandbag to keep the head straight. Place a third sandbag under the knees. This prevents strain on the knees and makes the baby more comfortable. Be sure the sand is evenly distributed and the hips are straight. Place a fourth sandbag over the knees and a fifth over the ankles if necessary. The lateral chest radiograph can be taken by immobilizing the legs the same way as for the anteroposterior view and holding the upper chest in position (Fig. 10–11).

COMMERCIAL RESTRAINING DEVICES

One of the more helpful options that come with radiographic equipment is the compression band. This device not only helps keep the child in position but also creates a safer environment (see Fig. 10–1).

The Pigg-O-Stat[5] is designed primarily for use in taking chest radiographs of children from 6 months to 3 years of age, depending on the size of the child. When you position a child for a chest radiograph, be careful to ensure that the hips are straight in

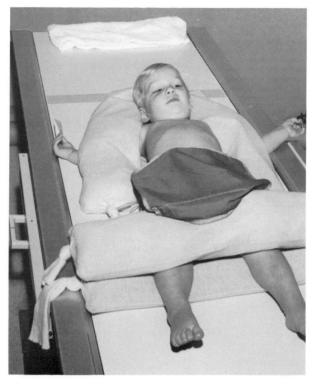

Figure 10–10
Child immobilized with sandbags for a recumbent anteroposterior radiograph of the chest.

the seat before you tighten the plexiglass sleeves, or the child's immobilized chest may be rotated (Fig. 10–12).

The Pigg-O-Stat works well for chest radiographs but can also be used for other examinations with some imagination by the technologist. For instance, it can be used for taking a lateral neck radiograph. Place the child's arms alongside the body and place

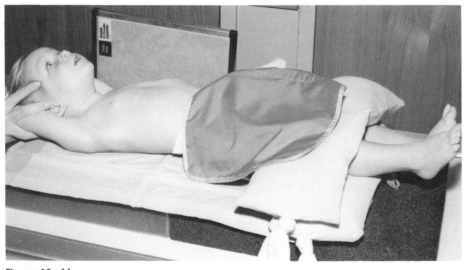

Figure 10–11
Child elevated on radiolucent sponges and immobilized with sandbags for a cross-table lateral radiograph of the chest.

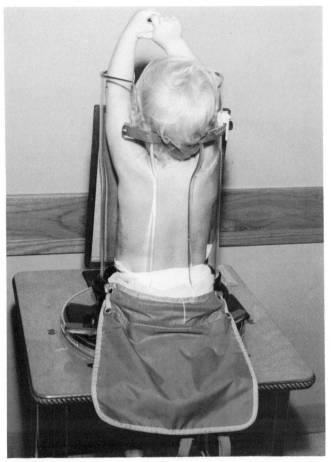

Figure 10–12
Child restrained in a Pigg-O-Stat (a commercial restraining device) for a posteroanterior radiograph of the chest.

a round sponge on each side of the head to immobilize the skull and ensure a straight neck.

For safety reasons as well as for immobilization purposes, infants under 1 year of age are radiographed supine. This can be accomplished with sandbags and radiolucent sponges, as previously described. Commercial restraining devices are also available, such as the one pictured in Figure 10–13. One company that supplies these is Contour Fabricator.[2]

The commercial devices cost as little as several dollars to as much as thousands of dollars. One important factor to keep in mind with all immobilization devices is that if they are not used as intended, they will not work. In addition, any device that is difficult to use will never be used by anyone. If the device is perceived as taking longer to prepare and position than does coaxing a child and struggling, the technologist will prefer the latter. A device that is not directly related to the child's size will not adequately immobilize the child. For example, when the table or base of the device is wider than the infant, the Velcro stretched across the child will not hold the child snugly because of the space created by the open angle.

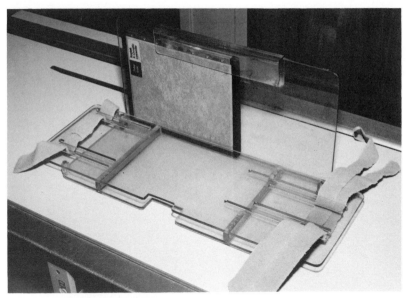

Figure 10–13
Commercial restraining device for immobilizing infants.

CUSTOM-DESIGNED IMMOBILIZATION DEVICES

At Children's Hospital we use several custom-made devices to help us immobilize children.

Chest and Torso Box. The film slides under the patient or is placed beside the patient for the horizontal ray lateral projection. The chest and torso box can also be used for decubitus radiographs (Fig. 10–14).

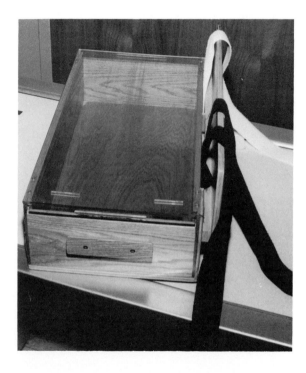

Figure 10–14
Chest and torso box for infants.

Chest Stand. A chest stand at the end of the x-ray table is used with children who are old enough to sit. It is important to tell parents that they may assist with the procedure. They should hold the child at the elbows, holding the head at the same time to avoid rotation. Velcro straps around the hips help keep the child more firmly in place (Fig. 10–9).

Seat for Barium Swallows. Our latest invention was devised to keep children still for modified barium swallows. Children undergoing these studies have problems swallowing and keeping still. Commercial products are available; however, none are suitable for children. The special seat allows us to fluoroscope children upright and keep them both secure and close to the image intensifier (Fig. 10–15).

Foot Boxes. To take radiographs of the feet with children standing, two boxes were made to stand on, one of which also holds the film. A parent must stay with the child for safety reasons (Fig. 10–16).

POSITIONING DEVICES FOR INTENSIVE CARE OR INPATIENT UNITS

If a patient is intubated, immobilization is probably not necessary. For infants who are able to move and need to be held in the appropriate position, restraining devices from the department or another bedside are not appropriate because of the possibility of transmission of bacteria or viruses.

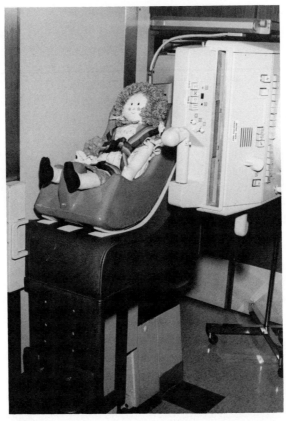

Figure 10–15
This seat keeps children secure and upright for modified barium swallows.

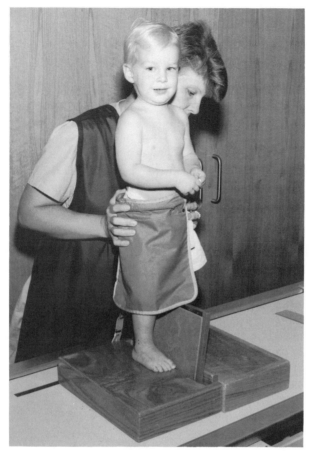

Figure 10–16
Foot boxes are used for standing lateral radiograph of the feet. One box holds the film.

To immobilize an infant wearing a T-shirt for a supine radiograph, unsnap the front, twist the shirt back over the arms, and secure the T-shirt to the bed with hemostats. Support the head in the correct upright position by placing rolled-up towels or blankets beside the head. Make sure that the endotracheal tubing is out of the way and supported by a towel to prevent it from snapping back into the field. Place a rolled-up blanket for support under the knees/femora to prevent a child who is semi-upright from sliding down. Pillows or blankets by their sides help hold older children upright.

Remember, no matter how many restraining devices you use, never leave the side of the child until you are absolutely sure that there is no way the child can escape the immobilization device and roll off the table or bed.

MANUFACTURERS

1. Johnson & Johnson Medical, Inc., P.O. Box 130, Arlington, TX 76004-0130, (800) 433-5009
2. Contour Fabricator, P.O. Box 56, Grand Blanc, MI 48439, (313) 695-2910
3. Chamco, Inc., P.O. Box 1268, Orlando, FL 32802, (407) 855-6636
4. E M Parker Co., Inc., 400 Research Drive, Wilmington, MA 01887-0540, (508) 658-0720
5. Modern Way Immobilizers, Highway 64 W., Route 1, Box 88, Waynesboro, TN 38485, (615) 722-3578

Preparation for Computed Tomography and Magnetic Resonance Imaging

MaryAnn Chin

WINTHROP-UNIVERSITY HOSPITAL
SCHOOL OF RADIOGRAPHY
MINEOLA, N.Y.

INTRODUCTION TO PATIENT PREPARATION

Computed tomography (CT) and magnetic resonance imaging (MRI) are two of the most sophisticated imaging modalities in a radiology department. CT and MRI use intricate computerized imaging systems requiring patient cooperation at the highest level to produce high-quality diagnostic images.

CT scan data are acquired by ionizing radiation, and MRI data are acquired by using powerful magnetic fields and radio frequency waves. CT and MRI are distinct and compatible. The decision to use one modality rather than the other or to use both is ultimately made by the radiologist. Referring physicians rely on the expertise of the staff radiologist to recommend the most appropriate imaging modality for a particular situation.

Unfortunately, many pediatric patients at the younger end of the age spectrum are uncooperative. This chapter deals primarily with the preparation of pediatric patients for sedation and the various methods of capturing a patient's attention before a decision is made to use sedation for a CT or MRI scan.

RESPONSIBILITIES OF NURSES AND TECHNOLOGISTS

The radiology department at Children's Hospital employs five radiology nurses. One is scheduled in the CT department and two are scheduled in MRI on a daily/weekly basis. The CT nurse works from 8:00 a.m. to 4:30 p.m. and handles all sedation and intravenous requirements.

The two nurses scheduled for MRI work from 7:00 a.m. to 3:30 p.m. and from 9:30 a.m. to 9:00 p.m., respectively. Patients are routinely scheduled for MRI during the evening shifts. Another radiology nurse is scheduled to cover the special procedures area, and the fifth nurse is the "float," with the responsibility of covering patients as needed in Nuclear Medicine and Diagnostic Radiology. The fifth nursing position was created to provide backup for vacation and sick-call coverage for the other nurses.

CT has two holding/sedation rooms, and MRI has three. The nurses working in each area play crucial roles in helping to maintain the flow of daily schedules for both.

The nurses in the radiology department at Children's Hospital rotate through all the areas that require daily nursing coverage, except the Interventional/Special Procedures suite, where the same nurse is always assigned. Daily responsibilities of the CT and MRI nurses include checking emergency equipment and making sure that all monitoring equipment is in working order. This includes checking the setups for oxygen and suction and the crash cart (life-support equipment) used for patient emergency codes. The CT or MRI technologist on call is responsible for maintaining and checking the emergency equipment if it has been used after 5:00 p.m. and on weekends.

The primary responsibility of the CT and MRI nurses is to evaluate, sedate, and monitor outpatients requiring sedation and to inject contrast media, when needed, through their cardiovascular lines.

Inpatients requiring sedation are assessed and sedated on their respective patient units. The floor nurses and house physicians have primary responsibility for sedating their patient for requested procedures. The CT and MRI nurses assume the monitoring responsibility for these inpatients only after they are brought to the department by their primary care nurse. The emergency room and intensive care units are responsible for the sedation of their patients, who are usually accompanied by the primary care nurse and the physician.

It is the responsibility of CT and MRI technologists to assist the nurses in their assessment of a patient's ability to cooperate for a procedure. The technologist decides whether to proceed with a scan or terminate the procedure on the basis of the patient's level of motion and/or cooperation. The main objective of a CT or MRI technologist is always to obtain optimal diagnostic images.

SCHEDULING SEDATION

At Children's Hospital routine CT examinations for sedated uncooperative patients or nonsedated cooperative patients are scheduled on an alternating basis. It should not be assumed that a patient will be cooperative based solely on age group.

Age is a chronological ranking, not an indicator of a patient's level of cooperation. The patient may be 8 years old and mentally retarded and therefore require sedation. One must always question the level of cooperation of all patients scheduled for CT or MRI. Some of the most difficult patients to scan are school age and older and are ultimately scanned using general anesthesia.

Patients are scheduled for sedation if there is any question or doubt about cooperation level. It is better to plan and schedule a patient for a more difficult and time-consuming procedure than to underplan and not be prepared should the patient require sedation.

One must factor in the time and effort required by the parents. If a return visit is necessary because the patient requires sedation for the procedure and was not properly scheduled, parents become particularly upset over taking another day off from work. The physician's appointment as well as the scan must be rescheduled. Another concern of parents is the need to arrange child care for the patient's siblings.

This scenario can be prevented if the person responsible for scheduling takes the time to look at the entire picture and accommodate the needs of the patient, parents, procedure, and physicians. If there is any doubt about the level of patient cooperation, the patient should be scheduled for sedation.

The most important aspect of scheduling patients is the communication of the sedation and examination preparations. The scheduling secretary, a very important link in the scheduling process, must be well versed and trained in giving out the proper sedation and examination preparation sheets. CT outpatients having abdominal scans must receive bowel preparation instructions.

The time requirement and the need for sedation are much greater with MRI than with CT. A routine head CT scan takes about 5 to 10 minutes, whereas the average head MRI scan takes between 20 and 30 minutes. The MRI unit at Children's Hospital has a day designated for general anesthesia patients on a weekly basis. MRI patients are more difficult to sedate as they must be kept sedated for a longer period.

The radio frequency pulses in MRI generate a loud, thumping noise, which awakens many patients. Thus, a stronger and more prolonged sedation may be required.

LEGAL ACCOUNTABILITY

In recent years there has been increased accountability for radiologists in their dictation of scans, for technologists in providing optimal scans, and for nurses in their judgment in sedating patients. Law courts have become arenas where staff radiologists are often called upon to provide expert interpretations of CT scans performed elsewhere, and where radiologists are accountable for interpretation of suboptimal scans.

As a result, CT at Children's Hospital has seen an increase in requests for more axial slices, more precise patient positioning, and additional views. This translates into an increased need to sedate patients. There has also been an increase in the number of complex disease processes, requiring more images and additional views, both axial and coronal, with and without contrast.

For example, patients with sinusitis had always been evaluated in the axial position only. The scan was performed by scanning 14 to 20 axial slices with 5-mm slice thickness by 5-mm spacing. Presently, patients with sinusitis are evaluated with coronal views and 5-mm thickness by 5-mm spacing as well as axial views.

Temporal bones were originally evaluated with 3-mm thickness by 3-mm spacing, bone algorithm, and 12 to 16 axial slices. Now requests are increasing for scans in the coronal position. Positive temporal bone disease has also increased; therefore, the need to scan before and after contrast injections in the axial and coronal views has also increased.

MRI has met with the same situation; the number of sequences requested by the supervising staff radiologist has increased. MRI requires continual upgrading of software; thus, more time is required to generate the upgraded sequences.

DIFFERENCES IN PATIENT PREPARATION FOR CT AND MRI

CT and MRI preparation is almost exactly the same for patients requiring sedation at Children's Hospital. The one difference is with bowel preparation for abdominal CT scans. Patients are required to take oral contrast the night before, 2 hours before, and 1 hour before the examination. The fourth and final oral contrast dose is given within 30 minutes before the scan, usually as the patient is getting on the scan table. MRI does not have the same requirement.

All patients scheduled for CT or MRI are required to be NPO (nothing by mouth) for 4 hours prior to the examination. The decision to give the patient a contrast injection is made by the supervising staff radiologist at the time of the examination. A nonionic contrast enhancement medium such as ioversol is used for imaging in CT, and gadolinium (Gd^{++}DTPA) is used for MRI. The dosage of contrast medium is determined by the supervising radiologist.

COMPUTED TOMOGRAPHY

CT SCANNING WITHOUT SEDATION

The most important aspect of scanning is establishing good communication with the patient prior to the examination. The technologist should introduce himself/herself to the patient and parent, explain the procedure, confirm the procedure to be performed, and chat with the patient. Ask patients old enough to comprehend for their version of the sequence of events and why they are having the procedure.

Ask whether this is the patient's first experience or a repeat procedure. The introduction should take place during preparation for the scan, before the technologists take the child and parent into the gantry room. Make explanations simple and clear, and never assume anything. You may be surprised by a patient's reaction or assumptions.

For example, the patient may have been told by "helpful" relatives that the examination is an hour long and that there will definitely be an injection of contrast. The fact is, we do not routinely give an injection for cerebral scans, and these examinations generally take 10 to 15 minutes. The child will have gone through a long period of needless anxiety by the time of the procedure and will be relieved to hear that there will be no injection and that the procedure will take only a few minutes.

Reassure the patient continually that the procedure is easy, and tell him or her the time it will take to complete the scan. Be truthful and straightforward. Children are intuitively aware of dishonesty. If an injection is to be given, let them know, using language appropriate for their age group.

Many CT patients at Children's Hospital are oncology patients and are seen on an ongoing basis—weekly, monthly, or yearly. It is important to develop a good rapport with these patients and their parents.

Although many patients live far from Boston, they insist on returning to our CT scanner and having the scan performed here. I have often asked them why, when they live closer to another facility, and they reply that they are "very comfortable with our technologists and feel a sense of stability and consistency."

At Children's Hospital the radiology nurse will feed a patient under 6 months old a bottle of clear liquids (such as 5% glucose water) in an attempt to obtain a simple cerebral scan without sedation. The success rate is high, and the images are of a very acceptable quality. Toys, stuffed animals, and rattles are available. The parents stay in the scanning room with their child and help to keep the child's attention. A familiar face and voice can make the difference in a successful procedure without the use of a sedative. Suspended from the ceiling is a colorful windsock and sparkling strands of stars and shapes. The constant flow of air from the ventilation system keeps the windsock and stream of glittering shapes in constant motion. This attracts and holds the patient's attention (Fig. 11–1).

Some parents are unable to hold their child's attention for a long period. The radiology nurse or a CT technologist remains in the scanning room, talking to these children. We ask parents to remain in the room during the procedure, as this helps a child remain calm long enough for the procedure to be completed.

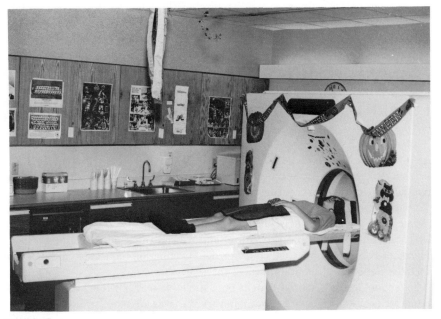

Figure 11–1
Computed tomography room at Children's Hospital, Boston, showing decorated gantry, windsock, and streamers, which attract and hold young patients' attention.

It is important to talk to patients of any age in the language they understand. Do not talk to an older child using baby talk or assume that a patient does not understand. At Children's Hospital a large patient population speaks Spanish. Language is an invisible barrier, and patients can request the services of a Spanish interpreter. Sometimes the interpreter is not always able to convey the appropriate information in a very short time, so keep talking to the patient in English, and maintain good eye contact. The sound of your voice, your gentle caresses across the chin and cheeks, and your smile are very reassuring.

A request for anything other than a simple, straightforward cerebral scan generally requires that uncooperative patients be sedated. The uncooperative patient may be a verbal 4-year-old child. The parent may insist on no sedation and plead with, beg, and then threaten the child to be cooperative. A young child may not be able to comprehend everything the parent is saying and may become more resistant and fearful. Although a simple, straightforward scan takes only 8 to 12 minutes, this period seems like an eternity to a 4-year-old, and a decision may be made to sedate the child. The decision is usually made by the nurse, but the technologist can step in and insist that the patient be moved from the scanning table to a sedation room and be properly sedated. It is in everyone's best interest to try to expedite the examination without upsetting an already frightened child.

BOWEL PREPARATION FOR ABDOMINAL CT SCANS

The amount of oral contrast mixture taken in the bowel preparation for pediatric patients varies with age. At Children's Hospital we use meglumine diatrizoate (Gastrografin) as the contrast medium. The dose is 10 cc of Gastrografin mixed with 8 oz. of juice, soda, or other beverage. All patients start with two doses the night before the examination and take additional doses 2 hours and 1 hour before the examination (see preparation sheet in Appendix B). The last dose is taken within 30 minutes before the CT examination.

If a patient requires sedation, the oral dosage is the same, and sedation is administered following the guidelines.

MAGNETIC RESONANCE IMAGING

MRI SCANNING WITHOUT SEDATION

First, MRI staff provide patients and parents with a checklist of specific questions related to the feasibility of qualifying for an MRI scan. The checklist is a safety mechanism to screen out nonacceptable patients—those equipped with such hardware as a cardiac pacemaker or Harrington rods.

As with CT scanning, the most important aspect is the process of establishing good communication. The technologist introduces himself/herself to the patient and parent, briefly goes over the scanning procedure, and asks if there are questions. Then the technologist reviews the checklist, confirms the examination requested, and determines whether the patient will be able to have the scan.

The technologist assists the patient onto the table and positions the patient using the required positioning devices, immobilizes the area of interest, and attaches the electrodes or grounding wires. The technologist continually reassures the patient that the procedure is painless and takes 15 to 30 minutes per sequence. The staff radiologist will decide on the sequences to be obtained.

PREPARATION FOR PATIENTS REQUIRING SEDATION

Until recently, there were only two methods of sedating patients for radiology procedures: oral chloral hydrate or intramuscular Demerol (meperidine) compound injection. Children's Hospital is in the process of changing to intravenous (IV) injection of Nembutal (phenobarbital) for patients over the age of 18 months and to oral chloral hydrate for patients under 18 months.

The department of radiology Sedation Committee is composed of an anesthesiologist, radiologists representing the different imaging modalities, a radiology nurse, and the technical director of radiology. The committee provides an atmosphere for a meeting of minds and demands acceptance by all members for a process to be approved. The main objective of the committee is patient safety and care.

Under the original protocol, patients were NPO for 4 hours before sedation. The new protocol, set by the Sedation Committee, required patients to be NPO for 6 hours. Parents voiced major concerns about keeping a child under 1 year NPO for 6 hours, and the Committee had to address these concerns.

Specific sedation protocol will not be discussed here, but it is important to explain the problems involved in revamping guidelines. Every institution has to go through this process for the above reasons. Institutions that sedate pediatric patients must follow guidelines established by their anesthesia department. This department must be involved in setting a radiology department's sedation guidelines, as the anesthesiology department is the group that responds to emergency situations caused by the sedation process.

At Children's Hospital, the department of radiology is currently using Nembutal as its major IV sedation agent. Hubbard and associates discuss the pros and cons of IV Nembutal in a 1992 article.[1]

The department of radiology Sedation Committee instituted the following preparation for patients undergoing sedation for CT and MRI:

Patients under the age of 1 year. IV sedation is not an option. The patient preparation is nothing to eat or drink for up to 4 hours prior to sedation. However, the patient may have clear liquids (including breast milk) up to 3 hours prior to sedation.

Patients 1 year to 18 months. IV sedation is not an option. The patient receives no solids by mouth for up to 6 hours prior to sedation. Clear liquids (including breast milk) may be given up to 3 hours prior to sedation.

Patients over the age of 18 months. IV sedation is used. The patient receives no solids for up to 4 hours prior to sedation. Clear liquids may be given up to 3 hours prior to sedation.

Patients requiring general anesthesia. The patient receives no solids from midnight the evening before the procedure. The patient may have clear liquids up to 3 hours before the procedure.

CT AND MRI IMMOBILIZATION TECHNIQUES

IMMOBILIZATION

Fold a doubled lengthwise sheet crosswise (quartered). Place the patient in the middle of the table. Fold the right end of the sheet over the right arm, then under the body, and pull to tighten.

Take the left end of the sheet and pull up gently, then across the right side of the body, and tuck the ends under the right side. The child is now in a mummified papoose wrap (see Chapter 10). Pull the restraining straps on the table tightly over the child, keeping the knees flat while maintaining a tight fit. If the child becomes highly agitated, try placing a large double apron across the body. If the child is still highly agitated, *stop*—this child is a candidate for sedation.

If the child has been maximally sedated and is still awake, lie across the child (who is still wrapped in full restraints), gently tap the chest, and talk in a very monosyllabic tone. I have put many children to sleep with my droning monologues. This is usually the last effort we make before terminating the procedure. We then reschedule the patient for general anesthesia. Fortunately, we have not lost many of these battles.

If being mummified has not agitated a nonsedated patient, give the patient a bottle of clear liquid, then scan the child as quickly as possible. Most patients (usually under the age of 1 year) can finish a 4-ounce bottle of 5% glucose water in a very short time.

The abdominal scan patient should be mummified and papoosed by the same method, but the arms should be raised over the head so a central venous line or peripheral line is accessible for the contrast injection.

THE 2-MINUTE RULE

If the nurse feels that a patient can be scanned without sedation, the patient must pass this 2-minute test. Hold the child's head in your hands for 2 minutes. If this does not bother the child, try to scan without sedation. Try the same method with the child in the coronal position (in the holding room) off the end of the stretcher. If the child passes the test, he/she is a good candidate for scanning without sedation. Our nurses are happy with this method of testing a child's cooperation level, and they can better assess the child's ability to hold still.

At Children's Hospital we scan all patients flat on the table, using soft foam head holders and sponges for positioning (Fig. 11–2). Velcro is attached to the sides of the

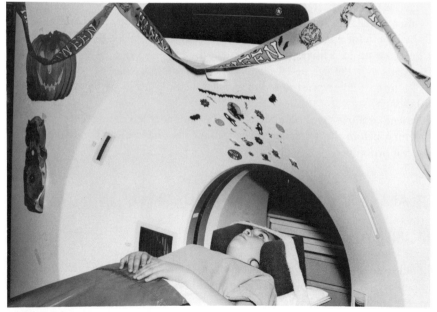

Figure 11–2
Soft foam head holder with a Velcro strap immobilizing a patient for computed tomography of the head.

table, and Velcro straps cross the table. This allows the child's head to be strapped very tightly into the foam head holder. We found that the commercial head holder was too high, too stiff, and uncomfortable for most younger patients. We have been scanning this way for 13 years and have not experienced any major artifact streaking or other problems.

CT VERSUS MRI

MRI scanning is very similar to CT scanning except that the patient requires a deeper level of sedation for MRI scanning. The MRI examination is longer and the noise level much higher. The constant loud thumping startles patients, and it is very difficult to calm the patient once the procedure has started.

With a 3- or 4-year-old child, the radiology nurse may decide to try the MRI scan without sedation. If a parent is willing and able, he/she lies on top of the child in the scanner and holds the patient's chin. Sometimes these attempts are not successful, and the child ultimately requires sedation. The radiology nurses always try to avoid sedating a patient needlessly.

Wrapping the sedated patient for MRI scanning is exactly the same as for CT scanning. However, the radiology nurse must monitor the patient with a pulse oximeter for MRI because the patient's respiratory rate cannot be monitored by direct observation.

The bore, or MRI tunnel/gantry, is deeper and narrower than the one used with CT. Patients tend to become somewhat claustrophobic in the MRI gantry, so the MRI technologist must spend more time coaching and reassuring the patient and parent that the patient will be able to handle the scanning process.

MRI uses different holders (coils) for the various procedures. The technologist confers with the supervising staff radiologist and receives a plan of scanning sequences and parameters. A radiologist is always present while CT or MRI scanning is in progress.

CT and MRI technologists who work with adults and whose stress level rises when they deal with an occasional pediatric patient should relax and have fun. Children know when the technologist is nervous, and this will make them less secure and more uncomfortable about having a scan. Talk to them and treat them with the same confidence you have with adult patients. You may have to refrain from using 10-letter words, but when you use simple language, they will understand what they need to know for the scan to be a success. Remember to be honest and straightforward at all times, and never promise what you cannot deliver.

SUMMARY OF SCANNING PEDIATRIC PATIENTS

1. Children under the age of 1 year can usually undergo a brain scan with mummified papoose wrapping while being fed a bottle of sugar water (5% glucose water).

2. If a child is verbal and has passed the 2-minute rule, proceed.

3. Sedation preparations are straightforward; the ultimate responsibility of writing orders for sedation on outpatients belongs to the radiologist. The referring physician writes the orders and gives the sedation for all inpatients.

4. Bowel preparation for abdominal scans consists of scheduled doses of contrast medium and does not alter the sedation process.

5. Technologists should be confident about their skills and remain calm when scanning children of any age.

6. Everyone should enjoy the experience. Children have no hidden agendas and are usually very compliant. They always want to do their best. Be honest. Joke with them. Tell them they are the best patients. Their smiles will light up your spirit.

REFERENCE

1. Hubbard, A.M., Markowitz, R.I., Kimmel, B., et al., Sedation for pediatric patients undergoing CT and MRI, Journal of Computer Assisted Tomography 16(1):3–6, 1992

Nuclear Medicine Imaging

Royal T. Davis

BACKGROUND

Pediatric nuclear medicine technology has experienced steady growth over the last 20 years. This is due in large part to advances in radiopharmaceutical development and instrumentation and, most importantly, the need to answer diagnostic questions related to pediatric disorders that could not be obtained or answered readily by other diagnostic methods.

The growth of pediatric nuclear medicine technology applications has been made possible by the ability to achieve early and improved diagnostic information with this technology. Nuclear medical diagnostic procedures are safe, minimally invasive, and sensitive, and they provide morphologic as well as accurate quantitative information about the function of organs and systems in the body.

Early on, pediatric nuclear medicine diagnostic procedures were mostly confined to children who were inpatients, were severely ill, or had cancer. The ability of nuclear medicine to aid in the early diagnosis of disease and to measure function had not been fully realized. This limitation was in large part due to the small radiopharmaceutical dose that could be administered and to instrumentation with poor spatial resolution. Most radiopharmaceuticals were tagged with radioisotopes with relatively long physical half-lives, resulting in significant radiation exposure to patients; also, early instrumentation allowed only limited quantitative data and images of low resolution.[1]

Advances in radiopharmaceutical research—particularly the development of pharmaceuticals labeled with isotopes with short physical half-lives: technetium 99m, (^{99m}Tc), iodine-123, thallium-201, and iridium-191m—have resulted in lower radiation exposure to the pediatric patient. Instrumentation has been developed such that cameras produce images of high sensitivity and resolution. The introduction of the digital computer to the imaging system has allowed recording and qualitative and quantitative analysis of studies. These major advances in the field have allowed for a shift in the types of pediatric studies requested. There has been a substantial increase in the number of studies for the diagnosis of benign disorders and in the evaluation of function. Also, the role of nuclear medicine in pediatric oncology is not limited to the diagnosis of metastatic disease; it has become more important in the area of early diagnosis and evaluation of disease.

TECHNICAL CONSIDERATIONS

The successful diagnostic pediatric nuclear medicine examination is a result of the proper combination of many factors, including the administered dose, injection technique, sedation and immobilization, imaging room, involvement of the patient's family, personnel, and imaging technique.

ADMINISTERED DOSE

Administered doses in pediatric nuclear medicine have largely been developed by experience. In most cases, absorbed radiation dose, photon flux, instrumentation, and examination times are the primary criteria in developing a recommended dose schedule. There is no perfect formula for pediatric dose administration. An estimation of a pediatric dose based on adult doses that have been corrected for body weight or surface area provides a guideline.[2] However, instrumentation and distribution of specific radiotracers in children versus adults must be evaluated when a dose schedule is devised. The biokinetics and biodistribution of radiotracers in the neonate are often different from those in the older child or adult. A dose schedule should indicate the minimum amount necessary to provide both a technically and diagnostically adequate examination.

INJECTION TECHNIQUE

Most nuclear medicine procedures require an intravenous injection for administration of the radiopharmaceutical. Therefore, the injection technique is very important, and preparation is the key to success. The technologist should prepare an absorbent, lined tray with all necessary items. This should include the labeled dose in a shielded syringe, saline flushes, gauze, disposable gloves, a tourniquet, tape, needles, and antiseptic wipes (Fig. 12–1).

The child is brought to the examination room and in most cases is injected in the supine position. (It is important that the technologist has enough help; many examinations require two technologists.) The site of injection must be identified. It is imperative that the site of injection not compromise the area to be examined. The patient's arm may need to be secured with an arm board or other appropriate device depending on age, cooperation level of the patient, and duration of injection. Once an appropriate vein is identified, a tourniquet is applied and the skin is cleansed. We recommend 25- to 23-gauge butterfly-type needles. The tubing is filled with sterile saline. With the help of someone securing the arm, the needle is placed in the vein. At this point, free flow of venous blood should occur, and the needle should be secured with tape. The tourniquet should be released and the needle and tubing flushed with saline (1 to 3 mL) to ensure patency before the radiopharmaceutical is introduced. If there is not free flow of venous blood and patency is questionable, another vein should be chosen.

For static imaging, the volume and speed of injection are not critical. However, for dynamic studies such as cerebral, renal, hepatic, testicular, or peripheral angiography, volume and speed are very important. In these cases a large peripheral vein such as that found in the proximal antecubital area is preferred. The volume of the radiotracer should be 0.2 to 0.5 mL, followed by a saline flush of 3 to 10 mL, depending on the age of the patient (newborn to young adult). A "T"-type connector with a one-way valve allows for rapid injection of the saline flush without interruption. It is also recommended that for imaging studies lasting 1 to 1.5 hours a small gauge intracath be placed.

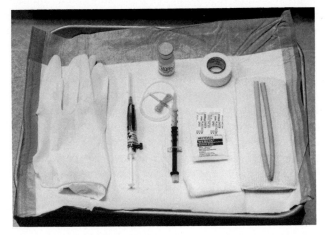

Figure 12–1

A tray prepared for the injection of a radiopharmaceutical. All the necessary items should be available to the nuclear medicine physician and technologist.

In the case of dynamic quantitative studies such as those associated with left-to-right shunt quantification and estimation of ventricular ejection fraction, a rapid and compact bolus close to the heart must be given. The antecubital vein in some cases may cause fragmentation of the bolus. In these instances, it may be necessary to use a deconvolution algorithm for the analysis of the study.

SEDATION AND IMMOBILIZATION

In most cases successful diagnostic procedures are done without the aid of sedation. In a vast majority of cases, technical skill, patience, time, and understanding result in a diagnostically successful examination without sedation. Less than 1% of our patients require sedation, and most of those require single photon emission computed tomography (SPECT) of the brain. Many of the patients referred for SPECT have seizure disorders and behavioral disorders that may require sedation because of the length of the procedure and the necessity that the patient not move.

In some cases it is necessary to use some restraint in lieu of sedation to maintain the patient's position for successful imaging. For these cases, sandbags, tape, papoose wrap with blanket, Velcro straps, and contoured pillows should be available. The papoose wrap is ideal for newborns. For older children immobilization with sandbags, Velcro straps, and tape is the norm. In all cases the patient should never be left alone in the imaging room.

It is important that all side effects associated with sedation be considered and that the imaging room be fully equipped to handle all possible conditions. Ideally, a nurse specially trained in imaging procedures should be readily available to the nuclear medicine department, working in conjunction with the nuclear medicine physician and technologist when sedation is required.

IMAGING ROOM

The imaging room for pediatric studies should be given careful consideration. The room and fixtures should be designed for the pediatric patient and should allow the nuclear medicine physician, technologist, and associated allied health professionals to care for the patient in the most efficient and effective manner.

Imaging rooms should be flexible in design so they can accommodate changes in technology. They should be quiet, comfortable, spacious, and attractive. They should have ceiling-mounted ambient light with dimmer switches, a wall-mounted examination light (which is useful for illuminating the area of injection or catheterization), a ceiling-mounted heating lamp, hangers for intravenous bottles, and a ceiling-mounted television set with video player. There should be a scale, monitoring equipment, emergency medicines, stethoscopes and sphygmomanometers for use with patients of all ages, and resuscitation equipment. Oxygen and vacuum outlets should be available and wall mounted. Ample storage space for all supplies should be available. The room should have air-conditioning. There should be enough electric outlets for computers, cameras, and additional equipment that may accompany the patient. There should be facilities for the safe disposal of radioactive materials and gases. The room should be situated close to the radiopharmacy for easy access.

Finally, the room should be equipped with all necessary communications: a telephone with cancelable bell and emergency numbers posted clearly, an emergency call button, and a silent security alarm. Provisions should be made for proper cabling to support all gamma cameras and computer systems.

INVOLVEMENT OF THE PATIENT'S FAMILY

The technologist should offer the parents their choice of involvement; some may choose not to be present. Some older children may prefer their parents not to accompany them.[1]

PERSONNEL

All personnel, physicians, technologists, nurses, and administrative support staff associated with pediatric nuclear medicine patients should be familiar with children and their needs, varied behavior, and disorders. Each pediatric patient must be looked upon as an individual with specific emotional needs. Pediatric nuclear medicine examinations are "people-intensive" and take approximately twice as long as similar adult examinations. More time and patience is required in dealing with the pediatric than the adult patient. It is recommended that more technologist and physician training programs in nuclear medicine include some training in pediatrics.[1]

IMAGING TECHNIQUES

Probably the greatest challenge to the pediatric nuclear medicine physician and technologist is the successful production of a high-quality diagnostic image. The instrumentation and associated hardware and software, if properly used, allow for this.

A very important diagnostic tool for the pediatric imaging specialist is the use of magnification, which, in its most proper sense, is the magnification of object size realized when using either a pinhole or a converging collimator. The pinhole collimator provides the best spatial resolution with the conventional gamma camera. The smaller the diameter of the pinhole, the better the spatial resolution. Other forms of magnification are called zoom. Both acquisition zoom and display zoom can be used with an all-analog camera and display system or with a computer-acquired and -displayed gamma camera image. Neither acquisition zoom nor display zoom can compensate for intrinsic camera resolution limit the way collimator magnification can, but in specific cases both play a useful role (Fig. 12–2).

The introduction of multihead SPECT has improved counting statistics and spatial resolution with reduced imaging time. This is a clear benefit when dealing with the pediatric patient. Early studies using zoom factors with multidetector SPECT have been promising (Fig. 12–3).

CLINICAL APPLICATIONS

The number of pediatric nuclear medicine examination applications continues to grow with newer and more organ-specific, short-lived radiopharmaceuticals and with the ever-improving instrumentation. The broad scope of imaging procedures for specific system evaluation includes the following.

NUCLEAR MEDICINE IMAGING PROCEDURES

Central Nervous System
▪ Brain scan and cerebral radionuclide angiogram

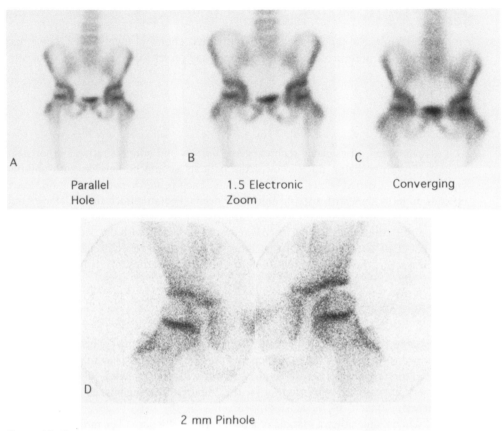

Figure 12–2
A through *D*, Images depicting different imaging techniques for evaluating the hip joint. The best resolution is achieved with the pinhole collimator with a 2-mm insert *(D)*.

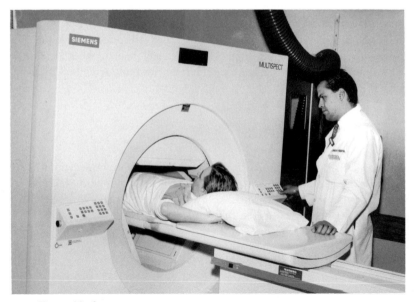

Figure 12–3
A pediatric patient undergoing a multidetector SPECT examination.

- Brain SPECT
- Cisternography
- Quantitative radionuclide cerebrospinal fluid shunt flow determination
- Regional cerebral blood flow

Cardiovascular System

- Myocardial perfusion (rest and exercise)
- Radionuclide angiogram for the evaluation of left-to-right shunts
- Venography/central venous line patency

Shunts

- Gated cardiac blood pool
- Cardiac SPECT
- First pass radionuclide angiography for the calculation of right ventricular and left ventricular ejection fraction

Pulmonary System

- Perfusion lung scan
- Ventilation and perfusion lung evaluation
- Detection of interpulmonary bleeding
- Radionuclide ciliary lung clearance
- Aerosol lung imaging
- Evaluation of pulmonary aspiration

Gastrointestinal System

- Gastroesophageal reflux and aspiration
- Gastric emptying
- Salivagram
- Salivary (parotid)
- Abdominal (Meckel's diverticulum)
- Hepatobiliary
- Liver spleen
- Detection of gastrointestinal bleeding
- Abdominal SPECT

Genitourinary System

- Renal vascular flow evaluation
- Renogram
- Evaluation of renal cortical defects
- Renal SPECT
- Diuretic renogram
- Radionuclide voiding cystography
- Testicular scan
- Determination of glomerular filtration rate

Musculoskeletal System

- Bone scan
- SPECT bone scan
- Intraoperative bone scan
- Bone scan for mandibular asymmetry

Endocrine System

- Thyroid scan
- Thyroid uptake
- Thyroid therapy
- Adrenal imaging

Lymphatic System

- Lymphoscintigraphy

Hematopoietic System

- Labeled white blood cells
- Labeled red blood cells
- Labeled monoclonal antibodies
- Bone marrow

Miscellaneous

- Dacroscintigraphy
- Gallium
- Gallium SPECT

COMMONLY REFERRED EXAMINATIONS

A few of the most commonly referred pediatric nuclear medicine procedures are described below.

Skeletal Scintigraphy

With the introduction of phosphates labeled with ^{99m}Tc,[3,4] pediatric bone scintigraphy has found a role in assessing numerous pathologies in the neonate, adolescent, and young adult. Among these are osteomyelitis, low back pain, stress fractures, avascular necrosis, osteoid osteoma, osteochondritis, osteosarcoma, Ewing's sarcoma, neuroblastoma, retinoblastoma, medulloblastoma, lymphoma, and eosinophilic granuloma.[5-7] The bone-seeking radiopharmaceuticals offer high photon flux for imaging, with an acceptable radiation dose to the patient.

Patients referred for bone imaging receive an intravenous injection of ^{99m}Tc methylenediphosphonate. At Children's Hospital the dose is prescribed by weight and is calculated at 7.4 MBq/kg (200 μCi/kg), with a minimum total dose of 18.5 MBq (500 μCi). Optimal imaging is obtained 4 hours after the radiopharmaceutical injection. A first-pass radionuclide angiogram (flow) may be employed.

Patients are routinely imaged in the supine or prone position; 500,000 counts (500 K) are obtained over the anterior chest, and the time is noted. In whole-body spot imaging, the remaining views are taken for that time frame. Additional imaging for the delineation of bony abnormalities may be done with SPECT or pinhole magnification scintigraphy (Fig. 12–4).

The importance of using the pinhole collimator (2-mm aperture) to improve spatial resolution in pediatric bone imaging cannot be overemphasized. An example of its usefulness is in the early diagnosis of avascular necrosis of the femoral head (Fig. 12–5). The initial decrease in uptake may be missed with the parallel hole collimator.

In some instances, three-phase bone imaging is indicated. This technique helps differentiate joint and soft-tissue disease from primary involvement of the skeleton,

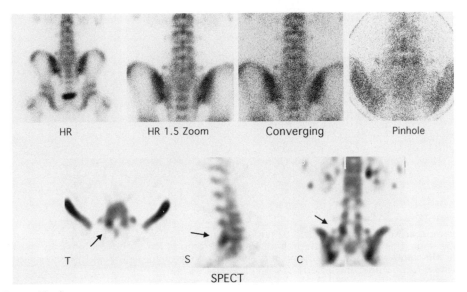

Figure 12-4
Different imaging techniques can be used to evaluate low back pain. Using SPECT, the patient's abnormality is noted in the transverse (T), sagittal (S), and coronal (C) images.

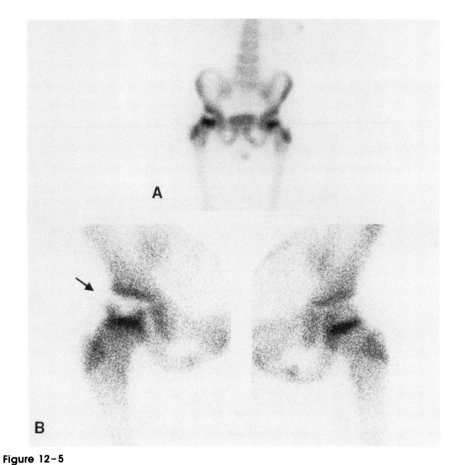

Figure 12-5
A, Planar imaging was performed on a patient who was referred for evaluation of the hip joint. **B,** Pinhole images show a lack of perfusion to the right femoral head *(arrow)*, consistent with avascular necrosis.

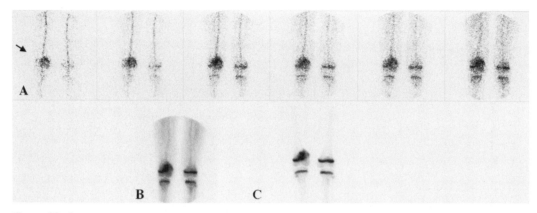

Figure 12–6

Three-phase bone imaging was performed to evaluate a patient's knee pain. **A,** The radionuclide angiogram shows increased blood flow in the area of the distal right femur *(arrow)*. **B,** The immediate static image shows increased uptake to the same region. **C,** The 4-hour image shows a focal area of increased uptake in the distal femur.

which is best seen in later images. Radionuclide angiography (the first phase) consists of one frame per second for 60 seconds, followed by a static image of the area of interest (second phase), followed by the later images at four hours (third phase) (Fig. 12–6).

Radionuclide Cystography

Radionuclide cystography (RNC) has a high sensitivity for the diagnosis of vesicoureteral reflux (VUR), with very low radiation exposure to the child.[8-13] RNC cystography is indicated for the initial diagnosis of VUR in patients with urinary tract infections (UTI), follow-up of known reflux, postoperative assessment, and evaluation of siblings of children with VUR.[14]

The direct method of RNC consists of a filling phase and a voiding phase. Bladder catheterization and retrograde filling of the bladder are required. The indirect method requires an intravenous injection and consists of a prevoiding phase and a voiding phase. Although good results have been obtained with the indirect method,[15] the direct method is generally preferred (Fig. 12–7).

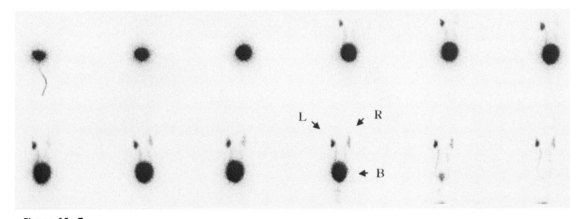

Figure 12–7

Radionuclide cystography, showing reflux on the left side (L) greater than on the right (R) at peak bladder (B) volume.

Direct RNC is straightforward. However, technical expertise is needed in dealing with the pediatric patient during urethral catheterization. Every effort should be made to explain the procedure in detail to the patient and the family. The child is asked to void before the examination. Catheterization is performed under aseptic conditions using a local anesthetic gel. Residual bladder volume is measured, and a urine specimen is sent to the laboratory for a bacteriologic culture. The patient lies supine on the imaging table, with the gamma camera positioned under the table to include the kidneys, ureters, and bladder. The study is recorded at a rate of one frame every 10 to 30 seconds. A radiotracer of 37 MBq (1 mCi) ^{99m}Tc pertechnetate is infused into the bladder and followed with a constant infusion of sterile saline. The infusion bottle should be positioned 70 to 90 cm above the level of the bladder. Infusion continues until the expected bladder volume is reached or the patient voids spontaneously around the catheter. The voided urine is collected and measured.

Reflux may appear at low bladder volumes, intermittently, during filling or voiding only, or throughout the examination (Fig. 12–8). Careful examination of the images as well as cinematic display of the study through its filling and voiding phases is very useful in the diagnosis of reflux.[13]

Renal Scintigraphy

Radionuclide evaluation of the urinary tract is important in the diagnosis of renal disorders and the evaluation of renal function in children.[16] These techniques allow evaluation of morphology and quantification of function simultaneously and thus provide information that cannot be obtained easily by other diagnostic modalities. The tracers used in these studies do not cause any toxic or even pharmacologic effects.

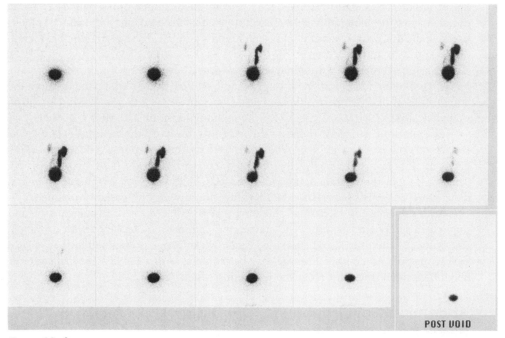

POST VOID

Figure 12–8
Radionuclide cystography showing bilateral reflux during the filling phase greater on the right side than on the left. There was no retention of the radiotracer in the postvoid image.

Unlike radiographic contrast agents, radiopharmaceutical administration does not provoke allergic reactions.[16]

Some common indications for pediatric radionuclide evaluation of the kidneys are hydronephrosis, pyelonephritis, renovascular hypertension, renal transplantation, multicystic dysplastic kidneys, and acute renal failure. Assessment of individual renal function and the dynamics of urine outflow is important in obstructive uropathy.[17]

Different radiotracers are used to assess renal perfusion, functional mass, and the excretory system.[18] Radiopharmaceuticals ^{99m}Tc-MAG$_3$ (mercaptoacetyltriglycerine), ^{99m}Tc-DTPA (diethylenetriamine pentaacetic acid), and ^{99m}Tc-DMSA (dimercaptosuccinic acid) are preferred.

Using ^{99m}Tc-MAG$_3$ or ^{99m}Tc-DTPA, imaging is accomplished in the posterior projection with the patient lying supine, using a high-resolution collimator. For patients with renal transplants, imaging is performed in the anterior projection. Urethral catheterization may be indicated in patients with suspected obstruction or reflux. The study consists of a radionuclide angiogram (one frame per second for 1 minute) followed by serial imaging up to 30 minutes (one frame per 15 seconds). If obstruction is ruled out early, the study can be terminated after 15 to 20 minutes. If obstruction is suspected, furosemide (1 to 40 mg/kg) is administered 20 to 30 minutes after the initial injection of the tracer or when the renal pelvis is filled with tracer. The study is then continued for another 20 to 30 minutes, and delayed images may be taken (Fig. 12–9).

Renal cortical function can be evaluated with ^{99m}Tc-DMSA. The patient is imaged 4 hours after the injection. Posterior high-resolution planar images are obtained with a calibrated radioisotope ruler to measure kidney size. Pinhole magnification as well as SPECT imaging may be used to delineate renal cortical defects (Fig. 12–10).

Scrotal Scintigraphy

Patients with testicular pain can be difficult to evaluate. Scrotal scintigraphy can be an important diagnostic tool when the clinical examination is equivocal and a decision must be made about whether surgery is indicated. Scrotal scintigraphy is useful in the diagnosis of epididymitis, epididymo-orchitis, abscess, late torsion, torsion of the appendix testis, or tumor.[19-21]

Imaging consists of a radionuclide angiogram followed by an immediate static image. Potassium perchlorate (6 mg/kg) is administered orally to the patient before the administration of ^{99m}Tc pertechnetate at a dose rate of 7.4 MBq/kg (200 μCi) with a minimum dose of 74 MBq (2 mCi) and a maximum dose of 370 MBq (10 mCi).

Patients are positioned supine on the imaging table, with the camera centered over the scrotal region. A converging collimator is used for the flow phase. The radiotracer is given as a bolus, and images are obtained every 3 seconds (128 by 128 matrix [computer acquisition parameters]) for 90 seconds. Following the flow phase, an immediate static image is obtained for 500 K while not moving the patient or camera.

After this image is taken, lead shielding is gently placed over the pubic region and thighs and under the scrotum. The converging collimator is replaced with a pinhole collimator (2-mm insert), slightly angled caudally. An image is obtained for 150 K (128 by 128 matrix). An additional image may be obtained with a flexible cobalt marker to help differentiate the right from the left hemiscrotum (Fig. 12–11).

Abdominal Scintigraphy for the Diagnosis of Meckel's Diverticulum

The detection of Meckel's diverticulum in the pediatric patient is important in the diagnosis of lower gastrointestinal bleeding. ^{99m}Tc pertechnetate concentrates in func-

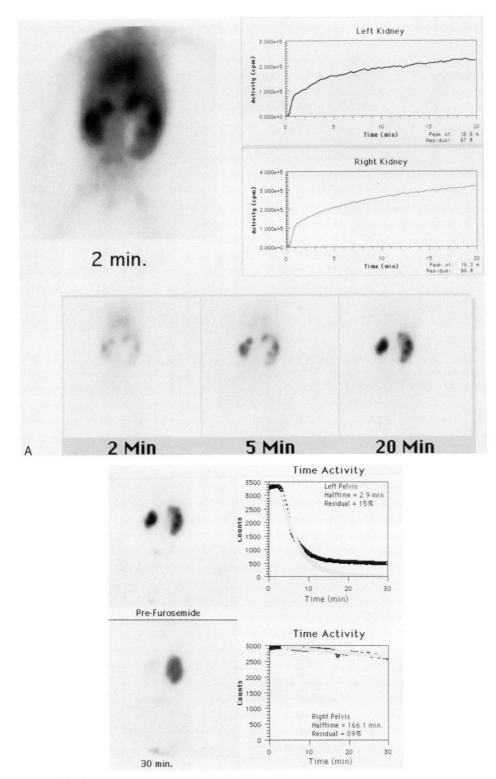

Figure 12-9

A, A renogram showing an enlarged hydronephrotic right kidney and a left kidney with a cortical defect. Both kidneys show delayed drainage, with tracer concentration up to 20 minutes. **B,** The diuretic renogram shows prompt emptying of the left kidney, with a halftime of 2.9 minutes and a residual of 15%. The right kidney has delayed drainage, with a halftime of 166.1 minutes and a residual of 89%.

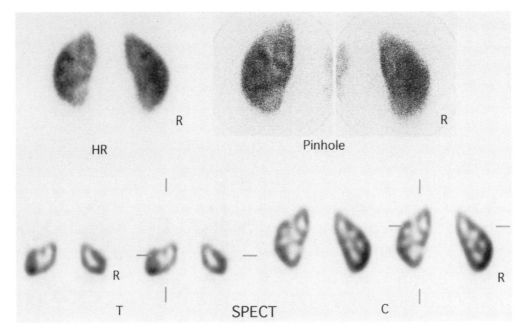

Figure 12-10

A DMSA renal scan showing a renal cortical defect in the upper pole of the right kidney. High-resolution planar imaging (HR), pinhole, and SPECT images were obtained. R = right; T = transverse view; C = coronal view.

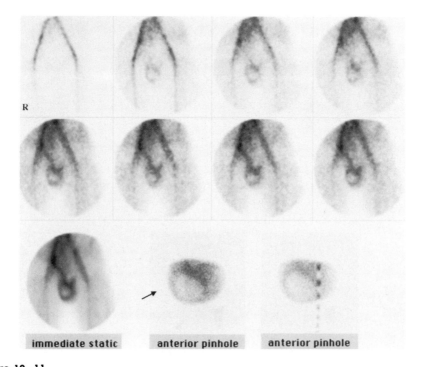

Figure 12-11

A testicular scan; the radionuclide angiogram shows increased tracer flow to the right hemi-scrotum surrounding an area of decreased flow. The immediate static image depicts a similar pattern. Anterior pinhole views show a photopenic area surrounded by increased uptake in the scrotum on the right, consistent with acute testicular torsion. R = right. *Arrow* denotes the "rim sign" associated with testicular torsion.

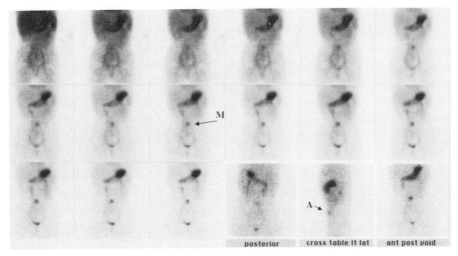

Figure 12-12
Technetium-99m abdominal scintigraphy from a 2-year-old male with a history of rectal bleeding. The study reveals a focal area of increased tracer uptake in the midabdomen (M) corresponding to ectopic gastric mucosa and Meckel's diverticulum. A cross-table lateral image shows the anterior location of the anomaly (A).

tioning ectopic gastric mucosa within a Meckel's diverticulum. Imaging with ^{99m}Tc pertechnetate is effective in the detection of such ectopic tissue.[22-25]

The patient should fast for at least 4 hours prior to imaging. No radiographic studies with barium should be performed before radionuclide scintigraphy, as the contrast agent may compromise detection of ectopic gastric mucosa by absorption of gamma radiation.

Pentagastrin (4 μg/kg) is administered subcutaneously 15 minutes before administration of the radiotracer. This enhances gastric mucosal uptake of ^{99m}Tc pertechnetate. The patient is positioned supine, with the camera centered over the abdomen.

The radiotracer is administered intravenously as a bolus injection and recording is performed at 1 frame per second (128 by 128 matrix) for 60 seconds, followed by imaging of 1 frame per 30 seconds for 30 minutes. Upon completion of 30 minutes of imaging, a cross-table lateral and a posterior image should be obtained. Also, it is recommended that a postvoid anterior image be obtained (Fig. 12–12).

THE FUTURE OF PEDIATRIC NUCLEAR MEDICINE IMAGING

Nuclear medicine imaging continues to provide important diagnostic information in the evaluation of pediatric disorders. With the advent of newer organ- and disease-specific radiopharmaceuticals and improved imaging technology, many pathologies not well defined in the past are now easily imaged. With the recent development of ^{99m}Tc-labeled brain imaging agents, assessment of regional cerebral blood flow and brain tumor activity is now possible (Fig. 12–13). Further, image registration technologies (now in early development) will increasingly facilitate the assessment of functional and anatomic relationships in the brain and other organs. For example, it is possible to "fuse" magnetic resonance imaging 3D image sets and SPECT of the brain.

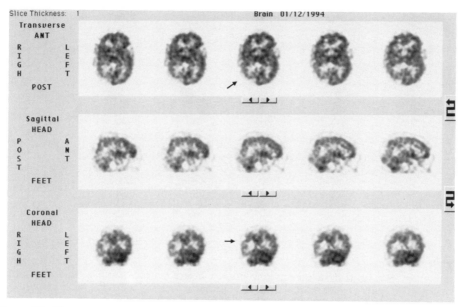

Figure 12-13

Selected transverse and coronal slices of perfusion brain SPECT (^{99m}Tc-HMPAO) reveal multiple perfusion defects involving the right occipital and temporal lobes (*arrows*). These images are from a 15-year-old male with focal seizures.

REFERENCES

1. Treves, S.T., Davis, R.T., Conway, J.B., et al., Introduction, in Pediatric Nuclear Medicine, p. xv, Springer-Verlag, New York, 1985
2. Cole, P.D., Espinola-Vassalo, D., and Alderson, P.O., Pediatrics, in Nuclear Medicine Technology and Techniques, 2nd ed., p. 523, P.R. Bernier, P.E. Christian, J.K. Langan, et al., C.V. Mosby, St. Louis, 1989
3. Subramanian, G., McAfee, J.G., Bell, E.G., et al., ^{99m}Tc-labeled polyphosphate as a skeletal imaging agent, Radiology, 102:701–704, 1972
4. Treves, S.T., Khettry, J., Brokes, F.H., et al., Osteomyelitis: Early scintigraphic detection in children, Pediatrics 57:173–186, 1976
5. Conway, J.J., A scintigraphic classification of Legg-Calvé-Perthes disease, Seminars in Nuclear Medicine 23:274–95, 1993
6. Harke, T.H., and Mandell, G.A., Scintigraphic evaluation of the growth plate. Seminars in Nuclear Medicine 23:266–73, 1993
7. Sty, J.R., Wells, R.G., and Conway, J.J., Spine pain in children. Seminars in Nuclear Medicine 23:296–320, 1993
8. Winter, C.C., Pediatric urological tests using radioisotopes, Journal of Urology, 95:584–587, 1966
9. Blaufox, M.D., Gruskin, A., Sandlee, P., et al., Radionuclide scintigraphy for detection of vesicoureteral reflux in children. Journal of Pediatrics, 79:237–246, 1971
10. Conway, J.J., King, L.R., Bellman, A.B., et al., Detection of vesicoureteric reflux with radionuclide cystography. American Journal of Roentgenology, 115:720–727, 1972
11. Conway, J.J., Bellman, A.B., and King, L.R., Direct and indirect radionuclide cystography. Seminars in Nuclear Medicine 4:197–211, 1974
12. Conway, J.J., Krighlik, G.D., Effectiveness of direct and indirect radionuclide cystography in detecting vesicoureteral reflux. Journal of Nuclear Medicine, 17:81–83, 1976
13. Willi, U.V., and Treves, S.T., Radionuclide voiding cystography, in Pediatric Nuclear Medicine, p. 105, S.T. Treves, Ed., Springer-Verlag, New York, 1985
14. Van den Abbeele, A., Treves, S.T., Lebowitz, R.L., et al., Vesicoureteral reflux in asymptomatic siblings of patients with known reflux: Radionuclide cystography, Pediatrics, 79:147–153, 1987
15. Handmaker, H., McRac, J., and Buck, E.G., Intravenous radionuclide voiding cystography (IRVC), Radiology, 108:703–705, 1973
16. Treves, S.T., Lebowitz, R.L., Kuruc, A., et al., in Pediatric Nuclear Medicine, pp. 63–104, S.T. Treves, Ed., Springer-Verlag, New York, 1985
17. Blaufox, M.D., Finc, E., Lee, H.B., et al., The role of nuclear medicine in clinical urology and nephrology, Journal of Nuclear Medicine, 25:619–25, 1984

18. Blaufox, M.D., The current status of renal radiopharmaceuticals, Contributions in Nephrology, 56:31–37, 1987
19. Nadel, N.V., Gilter, N.H., and Hahn, L.C., Preoperative diagnosis of testicular torsion, Urology, 1:478–9, 1973
20. Brodecker, R.A., Sty, J.R., and Jona, F.J., Testicular scanning as a diagnostic aid in evaluating scrotal pain, Journal of Pediatrics, 4:760–63, 1979
21. Vordermark, J.S., Buck, A.S., Brown, S.R., et al., The testicular scan. Use in diagnosis and management of acute epididymitis, JAMA, 245:2512–14, 1981
22. Jewett, T.C., Duszynski, D.O., and Allen, J.E., The visualization of Meckel's diverticulum with ^{99m}Tc pertechnetate, Surgery, 68:567–70, 1970
23. Sfakianakis, G.N., and Conway, J.J., Detection of ectopic gastric mucosa in Meckel's diverticulum and in other aberrations by scintigraphy: I. Pathophysiology and 10 year clinical experience, Journal of Nuclear Medicine, 22:647–54, 1981a
24. Sfakianakis, G.N., and Conway, J.J., Detection of ectopic gastric mucosa in Meckel's diverticulum and in other aberrations by scintigraphy: II. Indications and methods. A 10 year experience, Journal of Nuclear Medicine, 22:732–38, 1981b
25. Treves, S., Grand, R.J., and Eraklis, A.J., Pentagastric stimulation of technetium-99m uptake by ectopic gastric mucosa in a Meckel's diverticulum, Radiology 128:711–12 1979

Pediatric Ultrasound

Linda Sorensen
Cecilie Godderidge

INTRODUCTION

Ultrasound imaging uses sound waves to produce clinical images. Sound waves, like x-rays, transmit energy from one point in space to another, but few other similarities exist. Because sound waves are propagated by the vibration of particles in a medium, and particles do not exist in a vacuum, sound waves cannot travel through a vacuum. Whereas the velocity of x-rays is independent of medium, the velocity of sound waves is primarily determined by the medium through which they pass.

Sound waves are characterized by a number of different parameters. The frequency of the wave is the rate or speed at which the vibrating particles in the medium are oscillating. The common name for frequency in an audio system is *pitch*. Audible sound is determined by the frequencies detected by the human ear—approximately 20 to 20,000 hertz (Hz) (1 Hz = 1 oscillation per second or 1 cycle per second). Clinical ultrasound is performed in the 1- to 15-megahertz (MHz) range (1 MHz = 1,000,000 Hz). Because this frequency range is not detected by the human ear, the ultrasound scanner emits no audible sound waves.

The intensity of the sound wave measures the rate at which energy is transmitted from one location to the next. The common name for intensity in an audio system is *volume*. This describes the amount of force with which the vibrating particles move through their oscillations or the ability of the wave to do work. The intensity of the wave (expressed in units of watts/mm^2) is independent of the wave's frequency and velocity.

The characteristics of the medium in which the sound is traveling determine the velocity of the sound wave, independent of the sound wave's frequency and intensity. In general, maximum velocities are obtained in solids and smallest velocities are obtained in gases. Velocities through liquids are moderate. The average velocity of sound in soft tissue is 1540 m/sec. (1475 to 1620 m/sec., depending on the tissue's density). In skull bone, a solid, the velocity is 3360 m/sec. In air, the velocity is only 331 m/sec.

Reflection (change of direction) of the sound beam from interfaces between tissues in the body is primarily responsible for the production of the clinical ultrasound image. Ideally, a small fraction (<0.1%) of the incident energy of the ultrasound beam is reflected from each interface. This leaves plenty of energy in the original beam for it to continue to greater depths within the patient and to be reflected from deeper interfaces. If a higher percentage of the incident energy is reflected from an interface, the ultrasound beam cannot penetrate the tissue. This occurs clinically between the interfaces of greatly varying densities, such as between soft tissue and air or between soft tissue and bone.

In addition to reflections of the sound wave that remove the original energy from the beam, attenuation processes cause some of the beam's energy to be converted to heat energy. Because this lost energy does not make a contribution to the clinical image, attenuation needs to be minimized. Attenuation is directly proportional to the frequency of the transducer or ultrasound beam, so the lowest transducer frequency that produces an acceptable image will be the frequency that results in the most penetrating beam.

The ultrasound image is created by the detection of weak sound waves (echoes) that have been reflected from interfaces at all depths within the body. The machine simply maps on the screen the interface locations in the body. The strength of each echo is directly proportional to the depth of the interface from the surface of the body. The transducer of the machine uses electrical energy to vibrate a crystal within the transducer to produce the sound wave, which represents mechanical energy. The transducer's crystal is then quiet as it "listens" for the echoes to return. When an echo arrives, it causes the listening crystal to vibrate again. The induced mechanical vibrations in the crystal produce electrical energy. These electrical signals are used to determine echo depths. The weak signals are amplified and displayed on a monitor.

At first, only static ultrasound images could be created. Today, real-time images allow accurate imaging of moving interfaces. Doppler imaging, a more recent development, allows both the detection and the determination of the speed of moving objects within a stationary background, such as movement of red blood cells within the body's vascular system (see Suggested Reading for more information on ultrasound physics and instrumentation).

PREPARATION

Various approaches and techniques are needed (depending on the age group) to prepare children for an ultrasound examination. Although most examinations are noninvasive, the equipment, environment, and procedure are strange to a child. The darkened room, helpful to the ultrasonographer viewing the monitor, is often frightening to younger children. The procedure, the darkened room, and the use of the conductive gel should always be explained before starting the examination. The procedure may be outlined to the parent accompanying the child before they enter the room. A supportive and involved parent helps ensure a smooth examination. The less anxious the child, the more positive the experience and the better the result.

NEONATES AND INFANTS

Neonates and infants must be kept warm during the examination; newborns, in particular, become hypothermic very quickly. If warming lamps are used during the procedure, place them behind the equipment; otherwise the light from the lamps obscures the image on the monitor. The darkened room has a calming effect on patients in this age group, and a baby will lie quietly with the aid of a pacifier or feeding bottle. Warm gel and warm hands also make the study more tolerable. Light sustained pressure from the transducer is less disturbing than irregular contact, and the transducer can be held gently on the infant until the study is completed (Fig. 13–1).

PRESCHOOL AND SCHOOL-AGE CHILDREN

Preschool children tend to be afraid of the dark and may be sleeping with a night light on in their bedroom. If a patient is very frightened, leave a room light on even though it will be a little more difficult to see the monitor. It may also help to let the child hold a favorite toy or blanket. If a child will not lie down, suggest that the parent lie on the examination table with the child. In some cases, it may be helpful to let the child lie on top of the parent. If these strategies do not work, perform the scan with the child sitting or standing. For example, a renal scan usually performed with the patient prone can be done instead with the child standing and hugging his mother (Fig. 13–2). Be creative—do whatever is necessary to perform the examination.

All children benefit from having the examination explained to them beforehand, and constant reassurance should be given during the scan. Let the child participate by moving the transducer across his/her abdomen or by helping to smear on the gel. Show the child and parent the images on the monitor. Medical information regarding the diagnosis should not be given, but an explanation of the anatomy as the scan is being

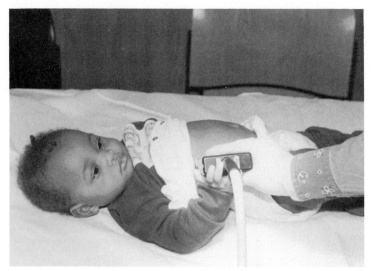

Figure 13-1
A transducer is held lightly on the infant's abdomen until the study is completed.

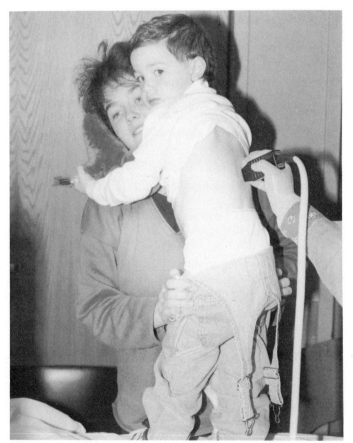

Figure 13-2
Renal scan performed with the child standing and hugging his mother.

performed makes the procedure more interesting and less frightening, particularly for older children.

ADOLESCENTS

Older children and teenagers also need constant reassurance, and their modesty should be respected. Keep the doors closed and the number of people viewing the procedure to a minimum. A scrotal examination is often embarrassing and therefore a difficult procedure for a teenage boy. We put a "Do Not Enter" sign on the door, and, if requested by the patient, a male ultrasonographer performs the scan. Ensure the same privacy for a female adolescent having a pelvic exam. Always ask, "Why are you having a pelvic exam?", particularly if the clinical indication is a positive pregnancy test. Other common conditions for a pelvic ultrasound examination for females include precocious puberty, abnormal menses, or assessment for ovarian tumor.

IMAGING TECHNIQUES

Differences in tissue attenuation are less in younger children than in adolescents or adults. There is less intrinsic fat, pediatric organs are closer to the skin surface, and the reflections from the interfaces are smaller in amplitude in younger children than in adults. Many different sizes and shapes of transducers are used, ranging from 2 to 7 MHz, depending on the examination and the age and size of the child. The most commonly used frequencies are 5 MHz, 3.5 MHz, and linear 5 MHz. The higher the frequency of the transducer, the less the penetration, but the greater the image resolution.

The operational modes used at Children's Hospital are real-time, including color Doppler imaging. Patients are scanned supine and prone in the transverse, longitudinal, and oblique planes. Transverse scans are viewed as if one were standing at the patient's feet looking toward the head. Longitudinal scans are viewed with the patient's head to the viewer's left and the feet to the viewer's right.

In most cases ultrasound studies are performed quickly, are noninvasive, rarely require sedation, and have proven to be ideally suited for examining pediatric patients. Ultrasound may be used, for example, in place of excretory urography in the investigation of urologic disorders, in place of barium studies in the diagnosis of pyloric stenosis, and in place of radiographs in infants with hip dysplasia, thus avoiding the use of ionizing radiation.

There are many clinical indications for ultrasound in pediatrics that are beyond the scope of this book. Following are a few of the more commonly performed procedures in the division of ultrasound at Children's Hospital.

ABDOMINAL ULTRASOUND

Indications for an abdominal ultrasound examination include abdominal pain, vomiting, weight loss, jaundice, trauma, and assessment for an abdominal mass. Fasting is frequently required to reduce intestinal gas. If an upper gastrointestinal barium study is requested in conjunction with an ultrasound examination, the latter should be performed first; otherwise the barium will obstruct the view of major organs.

Pain in the right lower quadrant of the abdomen may be indicative of appendicitis. A compression study is performed to show an inflamed appendix and/or appendicolith.

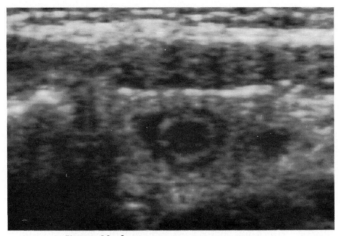

Figure 13–3
Transverse scan of an inflamed appendix.

If indicated, a plain radiograph of the abdomen is obtained before or after the ultrasound examination. A transverse scan (Fig. 13–3) shows an inflamed appendix.

Plain radiographs of the abdomen and chest should be obtained before scanning an abdominal mass. If there is abdominal distention, radiographs may show abnormal gas patterns and/or obstruction. An ultrasound examination should include determination of the organ of origin, the size and character of the mass, and the relationship to other organs and blood vessels; documentation of the adenopathy or metastases; and determination of vascularity.[1] Most abdominal masses in children are retroperitoneal, such as neuroblastoma; others are renal.[1] Other abdominal masses visible on ultrasound include liver tumors. Figure 13–4A shows a normal liver. Figure 13-4B shows a mass in the liver that proved to be a hepatocellular carcinoma.

During an abdominal ultrasound study in children, the abdomen and pelvis, including the bladder, should be examined. Transverse images are obtained in the following sequence: hepatic venous confluence, left portal vein, right portal vein,

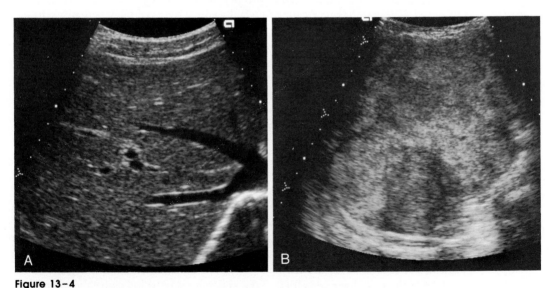

Figure 13–4
A, Transverse scan showing normal liver texture. *B*, Transverse scan showing a liver with heterogeneous echotexture, which proved to be a hepatocellular carcinoma.

pancreas, gallbladder, right kidney, liver, spleen, and left kidney. Longitudinal images include left lobe of the liver, aorta, inferior vena cava, gallbladder, right hepatic lobe, right kidney, spleen, and left kidney.

Cholelithiasis, common in adults, does not often occur in children. However, some conditions that predispose children to gallstones include sickle cell anemia, cardiac and orthopedic surgical procedures, cystic fibrosis, and anomalies of the biliary tract.[1] Figure 13-5A shows a normal gallbladder and Figure 13–5B, one with gallstones.

For a pelvic ultrasound examination, the urinary bladder must be full. The bladder assists in displacing intestinal gas and acts as an acoustic window to better reveal pelvic anatomy. Clinical indications in younger children include precocious puberty, a pelvic mass, pelvic pain, and ambiguous genitalia. Transverse and longitudinal scans are obtained to visualize the uterus and the right and left ovaries.

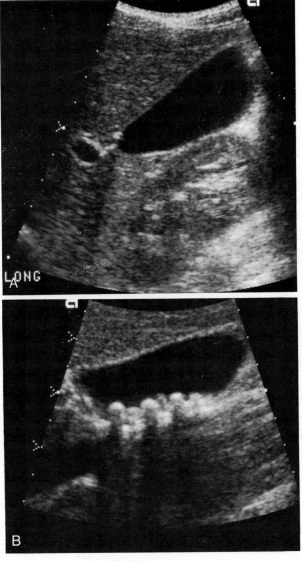

Figure 13–5
A, Longitudinal scan of a normal gallbladder. **B**, Longitudinal scan of a gallbladder with echogenic foci characteristic of multiple gallstones.

RENAL SCREENING

Renal ultrasound is one of the most frequently performed examinations in the department. Indications for renal screening include a family history of renal disease, prenatal diagnosis of hydronephrosis, abdominal pain, hypertension, painless hematuria, myelodysplasia, spinal injury, possible Wilms' tumor, and follow-up after genitourinary surgery.[1] The ultrasonographer must know the clinical question being asked when a patient arrives for a screening study and should recognize hydronephrosis, hydroureter, ureter/kidney duplication, renal stones, ureterocele, renal agenesis, polycystic kidney, and Wilms' tumor.[1]

Transverse, coronal, and longitudinal scans are performed to visualize the renal parenchyma and the collecting systems.[1] Figure 13–6A shows a normal renal outline in a longitudinal scan of the right kidney. Figure 13–6B shows hydronephrosis of the right kidney in a neonate diagnosed in utero. In scanning neonates and infants, the bladder is surveyed first, in case it is full, and before the cool air and the weight of the transducer cause the infant to void.

Ultrasound determines the anatomic structure of the kidney. If information about function is needed, the examination may be performed in conjunction with a radionuclide study of the kidneys or an excretory urogram.

RENAL TRANSPLANT

Renal transplantation is performed in children with glomerular disease, polycystic disease, and end-stage renal disease. Postoperatively, longitudinal and transverse scans are performed to evaluate the vascular supply, renal parenchymal echogenicity, and length of the kidney in these patients. The transplanted kidney is found in either the right or the left lower quadrant of the abdomen.

One of the most common reasons for an ultrasound study is to detect an increased serum creatinine level, which may be an indication of rejection. Figure 13–7 is a longitudinal scan of a normal transplanted kidney in the right lower quadrant with normal renal arterial tracing. Doppler tracings assess blood flow.

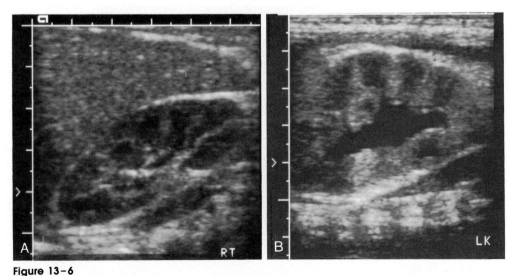

Figure 13–6

A, Longitudinal scan of the normal right kidney. **B**, Longitudinal scan of hydronephrotic right kidney.

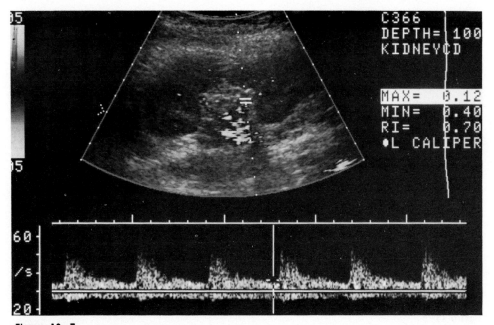

Figure 13-7
Longitudinal scan of a transplanted kidney in the right lower quadrant of the abdomen. Doppler tracing shows normal venous and arterial blood flow.

HIP ULTRASOUND

Ultrasound is now the imaging modality of choice in evaluating developmental dysplasia of the hip (DDH) in neonates and infants. As described in Chapter 8, radiographic findings may be subtle because the femoral head is not ossified at birth. On the other hand, the echogenicity of an infant's cartilaginous femoral head is well suited for ultrasound evaluation.

The infant is scanned in a decubitus position with the upper leg partially extended. The transducer is placed on the skin with its long axis in line with the ilium. Coronal and transverse images are obtained of both hips for comparison. Indications for this examination are a family history of DDH, asymmetrical hip creases, breech birth, hip "clicks," and feet anomalies. Coronal scans show a normal right hip in Figure 13–8A and a dislocated left hip in Figure 13–8B.

PYLORIC STENOSIS

Indications for a pyloric stenosis ultrasound examination are nonbilious projectile vomiting and weight loss. The etiology (as discussed in Chapter 3) is obscure, but it is an anomaly in which the pyloric muscle is thickened and the canal becomes elongated and narrow. An olive-shaped mass palpated during clinical examination may be seen as a soft-tissue shadow on a plain radiograph of the abdomen.

The infant is placed in a right posterior oblique position to encourage distention of the pyloric antrum with fluid.[1] The gallbladder is a useful landmark, as it tends to overlie the duodenal cap. The transducer is placed on the abdomen so that its long axis is aligned with the pyloric canal. Muscle thickness and length of the channel are measured. Figure 13–9 shows a thickened, elongated pyloric muscle in a patient with pyloric stenosis.

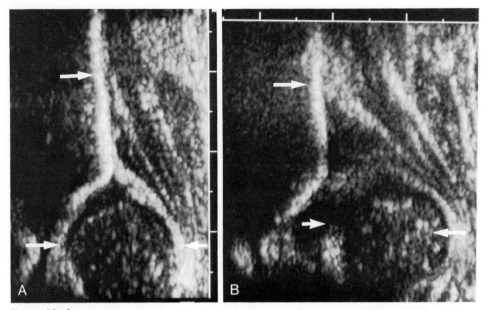

Figure 13-8

A, Normal right hip. Coronal scan shows the iliac bone line (*arrow*) bisecting the femoral head. The cartilaginous femoral head (*between arrowheads*) is positioned normally. *B*, Abnormal right hip. Coronal scan shows complete dislocation of the right hip. The femoral head (*between arrowheads*) is laterally displaced away from the acetabulum. In this case, the iliac bone line (*arrow*) does not bisect the femoral head.

CRANIAL ULTRASOUND

Cranial ultrasound of premature babies is usually performed in the neonatal intensive care unit because it is easier to take the equipment to a sick baby than to transport the baby. Cleanliness is important; special care should be taken to ensure that the transducer is clean and the technologist's hands are well scrubbed and/or gloved before the examination. The ultrasonographer should also ensure that the baby is kept warm throughout the examination.

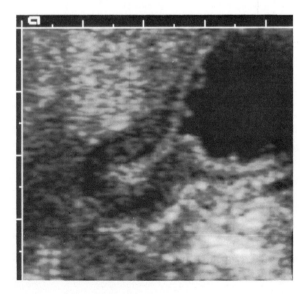

Figure 13-9

Longitudinal scan shows a thickened, elongated pyloric muscle, diagnostic of pyloric stenosis. The adjacent echolucent structure is the fluid-filled stomach.

Screening for intracranial hemorrhage is a common request from the newborn nursery because premature babies are at a higher risk for bleeds. Six standard views are performed in the coronal planes: orbital roofs, pentagon view (circle of Willis), third and fourth ventricles, trigones, and over the top of the lateral ventricles. Six standard views are performed in the sagittal plane: two midline views, and two parasagittal views of the right and left sides of the brain.

Figure 13–10*A* is a sagittal midline view of the brain; Figure 13–10*B* is a coronal scan of the pentagon view. The pentagon is a five-pointed star formed by the internal carotid artery, middle cerebral artery, anterior communicating arteries, anterior horns of lateral ventricles, genu of the corpus callosum, basal ganglia, subependymal germinal matrix, and tips of the temporal lobes.[1]

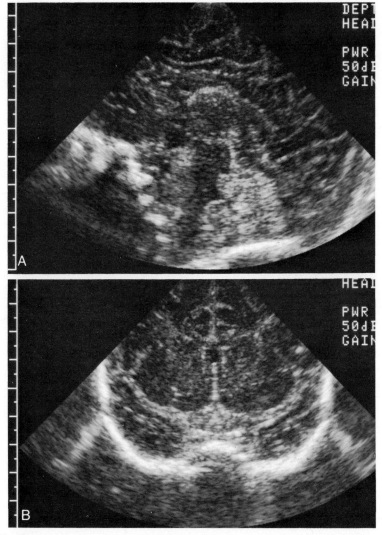

Figure 13–10
A, Sagittal scan of a neonate brain showing normal midline structures. *B*, Coronal scan showing pentagon view of a normal neonate brain.

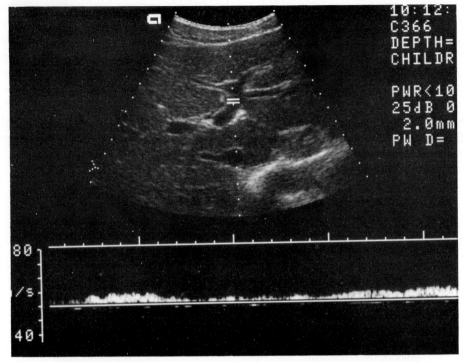

Figure 13–11
Doppler image of the portal vein showing normal blood flow into the liver (hepatopetal—tracing above the baseline).

PULSED DOPPLER

Echoes reflected from stationary interfaces are weaker than the sound waves that enter the patient, but they have the same frequency. In contrast, if interfaces move relative to the transducer, the echoes also undergo a change in frequency. In 1842, Christian Johann Doppler observed that the wavelength of light varies according to the relative motion of the source and the observer.[2] The same effect is also true of sound waves, and changes in frequency between the original ultrasound beam and the echoes reflected from the moving object or substance are used to image blood flow. Pulsed Doppler and color Doppler ultrasound are used to evaluate the direction and velocity of blood flow in, for example, patients with liver and renal transplants, hepatomegaly, splenomegaly, scrotal masses, deep-vein thrombosis, and to evaluate the vascularity of a mass or lesion. Figure 13–11 shows Doppler tracing of normal blood flow through the portal vein.

REFERENCES

1. Teele, L.T., and Share, J.C., Ultrasonography of Infants and Children, W.B. Saunders Company, Philadelphia, 1991
2. Bushong, S.C., Radiologic Science for Technologists, 5th ed., C.V. Mosby, St. Louis, 1993

SUGGESTED READING

Hykes, D.L., Hedrick, W.R., and Starchman, D.E., Ultrasound Physics and Instrumentation, 2d ed., C.V. Mosby, St. Louis, 1992

Chapter 14

Radiation Protection in Children

INTRODUCTION

The cumulative effects of radiation and the potential for harm is greater for children than for adults because of children's life expectancy, the frequency of some radiologic procedures, and the radiosensitivity of rapidly dividing cells. Many childhood diseases require follow-up imaging even into adulthood, and every effort should be made to minimize radiation dosage.

Children are a mass of growing, changing cells. They are considered biologically more sensitive to radiation, and protection should always be a consideration in any procedure. Radiation dose to children is lower than to adults because children are smaller, but as radiographers, we have a responsibility to keep the dose as low as reasonably achievable, particularly to critical organs that may be more radiosensitive than those of adults.

Stochastic and nonstochastic effects are the two general categories of radiation-induced diseases. Nonstochastic describes a somatic effect directly related to radiation exposure, in which the severity increases with the level of absorbed dose.[1] The higher the dose, the greater the damage, which is mainly degenerative, such as lens opacification.

A stochastic effect is a random, all-or-none response that may or may not arise because of radiation injury to a single cell or gene.[1] Malignant tumors, leukemia, and genetic effects are considered the main stochastic effects of exposure to lower levels of ionizing radiation.[1] Radiation protection guidelines for diagnostic radiology assume a linear nonthreshold dose-risk relationship, and therefore any radiation dose — small or large — is expected to produce a response.

Studies of atom bomb survivors have shown that the lifetime risk of carcinogenic effects varies with the age of the individual at the time of exposure. The National Research Council, in its fifth report on the biological effects of ionizing radiation (BEIR V), states that cancer risks from radiation exposure during childhood are estimated to be about double that during adulthood, although continued monitoring of the Japanese atom bomb survivors will be necessary to confirm this estimate.[2] The risk of radiogenic breast cancer is greatest from exposure during adolescence, according to follow-up studies of patients with pulmonary tuberculosis whose treatment between 1930 and 1954 included frequent chest fluoroscopy.[3,4]

There are two specific objectives of radiation protection: (1) to prevent, as far as practicable, the occurrence of severe radiation-induced nonstochastic diseases by adhering to dose-equivalent limits that are below the apparent practical threshold dose-equivalent levels and (2) to limit the risk of stochastic effects, fatal cancer, and genetic effects to a reasonable level compared with nonradiation risks and in relation to society's needs, benefits gained, and economic factors.[1]

To limit children's exposure to radiation it is essential that radiographers be trained in pediatric radiology. In order to minimize repeat radiographic studies, children should be properly positioned and immobilized, a minimal number of films should be taken, and appropriate exposure factors should be chosen. Exact collimation is essential, and when a body part particularly sensitive to radiation is in the primary beam, protective lead shielding or alternative positioning (posteroanterior versus anteroposterior, as described for the complete spine [see Chapter 7]) should be used. This, of course, assumes that the area of diagnostic interest is not obscured by the shield.

GONADAL SHIELDING

To limit genetic effects, gonadal shielding should be used if the testes or ovaries are in the direct x-ray beam or close to the edge of the collimated area. Generally, it is easier to shield the male testes because they are outside the body cavity. A contact shield over the testes reduces radiation exposure by about 95%[5] (Fig. 14–1). Ovarian shielding, although more complex because of the variability in the location of the ovaries, can reduce exposure by up to 50%[5] (Fig. 14–2).

A gonad shielding protocol should be established for all routine procedures; the protocol may be a simple chart similar to the one at the end of Appendix C. At Children's Hospital we do not use a gonadal shield for a first examination of the hips or pelvis, but one is required on follow-up radiographs as long as the shield does not cover the site of a previous surgical procedure.

There are several types of lead gonadal shields. One is a shadow shield, which is attached to the x-ray tube or the side of the collimator. The shield is moved into place in front of the collimator to block the x-ray beam. The shield does not touch the patient, so hygiene is not an issue; it can also be used in a sterile field. Another advantage is that it is easier to keep the shield in position when a patient is standing. The shields are supplied in one size or a multiple pattern to accommodate male and female patients of different sizes. It is difficult to maintain the correct shadow placement on infants and younger children, who are more difficult to immobilize.

Another type is the contact shield, which is placed on the patient. Contact shields can be purchased or made in a variety of shapes and sizes and are better for children, as it is easier to accommodate the various sizes of patients. At Children's Hospital we make our own shields from 1-mm lead vinyl sheeting for both male and female patients. Lead shields for males are shaped in four graduated sizes: very small, small, medium, and large (Fig. 14–3). The sizes are estimated and are not based on any specific measurements.

A study was done at Children's Hospital in the late 1970's to assess the range of sizes needed for the female patients because of the inherent difficulties in shielding the

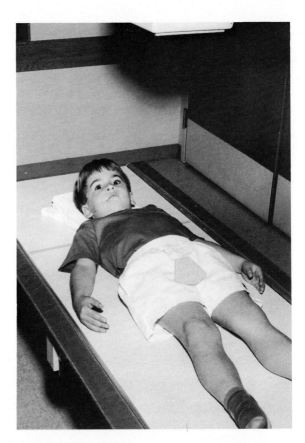

Figure 14–1
Shaped contact shield covering the testes.

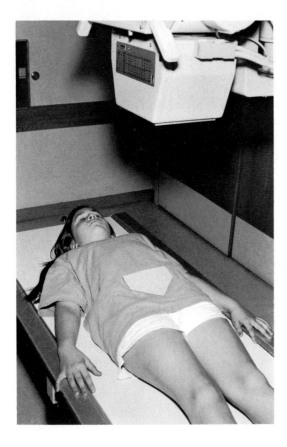

Figure 14-2
Shield designed at Children's Hospital, Boston, for covering the ovaries.

ovaries. Figure 14-4 shows the variations that can occur in the location of the ovaries from 1 day to 12 years. Thirty females of different ages and sizes were measured from the inner aspect of one anterior superior iliac spine to the other and from the center of this line to the upper border of the symphysis pubis.[6]

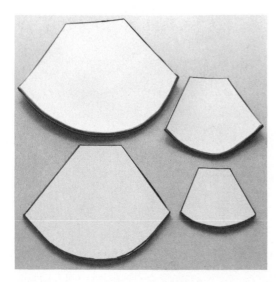

Figure 14-3
Various shapes of 1-mm lead vinyl shields for males (actual size not shown).

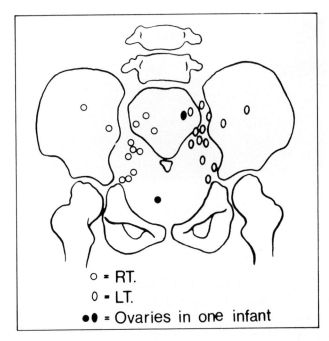

Figure 14-4
Diagram showing the variation at pathology in the location of the female ovaries from 1 day to 12 years. RT = right; LT = left. (From D'Angio, G.J., and Tefft, M., Radiation therapy in the management of children with gynecologic cancers, Annals of the New York Academy of Sciences, 142:675–693, 1967.)

From these measurements, five graduated sizes that would cover most conditions and age groups were chosen (Fig. 14–5):[6]

13 years to adult	y = 18 cm	x = 7 cm
10 to 13 years	y = 14 cm	x = 7 cm
7 to 9 years	y = 12 cm	x = 7 cm
3 to 6 years	y = 12 cm	x = 4 cm
3 months to 2 years	y = 8 cm	x = 4 cm

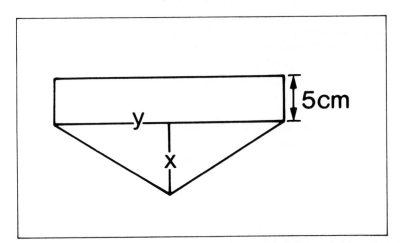

Figure 14-5
Gonadal shield template showing the base extended to absorb scatter radiation from the edge of the field. (From Godderidge, C., Female gonadal shielding, Applied Radiology, 8(2):65–67, 1979.)

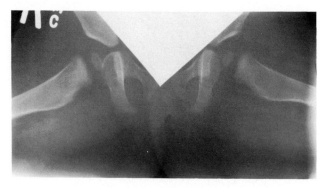

Figure 14-6
Radiograph of both hips showing accurate placement of the ovarian shield.

Templates were made from stiff card material, and because the shields were to be used for hip examinations, the sides were cut at a steep angle from the apex to the base of the triangle, to avoid the hip joints. The base of the triangle was extended to 5 cm at the recommendation of our physicist because of the estimated falloff of approximately 20% in scatter radiation 1 cm from the edge of the field[6] (see Fig. 14–5). The shield would then also cover ovaries situated higher in the pelvic cavity.

The line "y" drawn on the shield should be level with the anterior superior iliac spines and the apex of the triangle on the upper border of the symphysis pubis. This shield is not easy to use, but when positioned correctly, it will cover most of the pelvic area without obscuring the hip joints (Fig. 14–6). It may not be suitable for patients who have had surgical reconstruction around the ilium and acetabulum. Radiographers should carefully check the patient's clinical history and previous x-rays before placing the shield.

Shielding of any kind is difficult on female newborns and infants. The abdomen is round and mobile; the upper parts of the legs have folds, and it is difficult to palpate the symphysis pubis. It is also difficult to maintain the position of the shield, which may slip, obscuring the hip joints. If more than one view is taken, it is suggested that the patient be shielded on one film only. Fortunately, fewer radiologic hip examinations are performed today on infants for congenital dislocation of the hip, as most cases are diagnosed by ultrasound.

A shaped contact shield is another type of gonadal shield for males. These shields are not very popular because some female radiographers are reluctant to use them, patient hygiene is a concern, and appropriate underpants are needed to hold the shield. These shields are useful for fluoroscopic procedures when other types of shielding are ineffective.

The male testes can be shielded on most examinations of the abdomen and pelvis if the urethra is not being evaluated. The ovaries can be shielded for examinations of the hips but not when the lower abdomen or pelvis needs to be visualized. At Children's Hospital we do not routinely shield patients who have been diagnosed with metastases or pelvic trauma.

PROTECTIVE APRONS

Protective half-aprons (sometimes called mini-aprons or demi-aprons) are sold in a variety of sizes to fit patients of all ages (Fig. 14–7). They are usually supplied with a

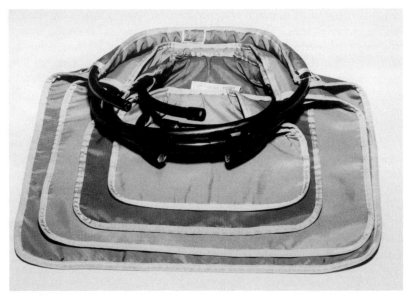

Figure 14-7
Half-aprons made of 0.5-mm lead equivalent come in four sizes. (Manufactured by Burkhart Roentgen, Cornwall Bridge, CT, and Bar-Ray Products, Inc., Brooklyn, New York.)

storage rack in sets of four. An apron can be placed on a child or fastened around the waist for examinations of the chest or extremities. For upright films, adjustable waist-high mobile shields can be used on older children.

These protective shields should never be used in lieu of precise collimation. Most are constructed of 0.5-mm lead equivalent, which will not completely absorb primary beam. Half-aprons are for the absorption of scatter radiation and to help protect the gonads, particularly when the gonads are close to the area under examination.

THYROID SHIELDING

The National Council on Radiation Protection and Measurement report titled *Radiation Protection in Pediatric Radiology* states that shielding the thyroid is not practical in most radiologic examinations. With chest examinations it is not possible, because visualization of the airway in the neck is often important.[7]

Because of concerns about the number of chest radiographs obtained on premature infants and the consequent radiation to the thyroid, some years ago we tried to devise a lead thyroid collar for neonates. These patients are radiographed supine; the projection is anteroposterior, so the thyroid receives almost the equivalent of the skin entrance radiation dose. The collar, however, though protecting the thyroid, obscured the neck and apices. Follow-up studies estimated the entrance dose to the chest at less than 5 mrad (0.005 cGy) on these small infants, so the overall cumulative dose to the thyroid was not as high as was originally believed.

BREAST SHIELDING

Studies in the late 1970's of Japanese atom bomb survivors, women with tuberculosis who were frequently examined fluoroscopically, and women irradiated for postpartum mastitis determined that age at exposure is a major influence in the development of breast cancer.[3,4] These studies provided strong evidence for cancer induction in females who were exposed at ages 10 to 19, 20 to 29, and 30 to 39; those 10 to 19 years of age had the greatest risk.[3] "These findings underscored the importance of hormonal influences on radiogenic breast cancer risk and suggest that proliferating tissue during the time of breast budding or pregnancy may be particularly sensitive to ionizing radiations."[3]

The results of this study and other similar studies convinced us to change our protocol of radiographing the complete spine for the evaluation of scoliosis from an anteroposterior to the posteroanterior projection. When the patient faces the film, the breasts receive the exit dose rather than the skin entrance radiation dose (Fig. 14-8). We also use a wedge filter to even out the density in the cervicothoracic region and a 1200-speed screen/film system.

Even though we have followed this procedure for many years, more recently breast shielding has been requested by parents and their daughters. The lead drapes shown in the literature from commercial suppliers are protecting patients whose spines are straight. For those with scoliosis, particularly if it is severe, the curvature may be obscured by a lead drape or shawl. We tried placing pieces of lead in the appropriate position on the patient's back, but they were difficult to tape in place.

Presently we use a compensation wedge filter system to which lead breast shields can be attached magnetically to one or both sides of the device (Fig. 14-9). The shields are easily visualized in the light field, and correct placement is simple with a little practice. These shields can be used for both posteroanterior and lateral projections of the spine.

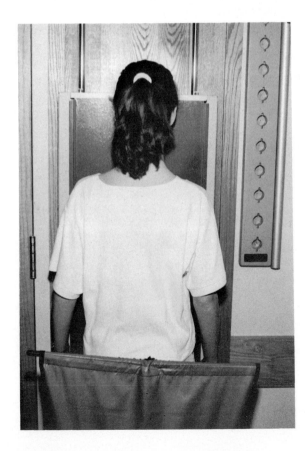

Figure 14-8

A patient stands facing an upright 3-foot cassette stand for a posteroanterior radiograph of the spine from C1 to S2 in the evaluation of scoliosis. Breasts (without shielding) receive the exit dose rather than the entrance dose.

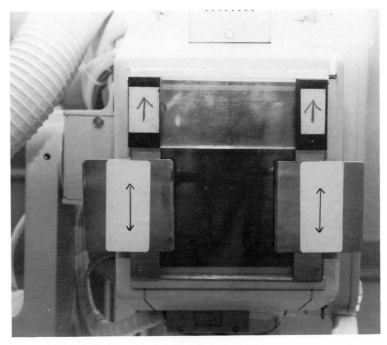

Figure 14-9
A patient protection system with a wedge compensation filter and magnetically mounted breast shields. (Manufactured by Nuclear Associates, Division of Victoreen, Inc., Carle Place, New York.)

LENS SHIELDING

Whenever possible, the skull should be radiographed posteroanteriorly rather than anteroposteriorly to reduce radiation exposure to the lens. This is not very practical with children because they are less frightened by a procedure when they can see what is going on around them. Eye shields have been used, but in most cases they obscure the area of clinical interest or, as in computed tomography, appear as artifacts.

Fewer routine radiologic examinations of the skull are being performed since the advent of computed tomography and magnetic resonance imaging. Multidirectional tomography, which was responsible for a comparatively high dose of radiation to the lens, has largely been replaced by newer technology. Most of our skull examinations are for sinuses, and it is preferable to radiograph the skull posteroanteriorly rather than anteroposteriorly so that the lens will receive the exit dose rather than the skin entrance radiation dose.

REFERENCES

1. National Council on Radiation Protection and Measurements, Report No. 91, Recommendations on Limits for Exposure to Ionizing Radiation, National Council on Radiation Protection and Measurements, Bethesda, MD, 1987
2. National Research Council. Health Effects of Exposure to Low Levels of Ionizing Radiation. BEIR V. Washington, DC. National Academy Press, 1990
3. Boice, J.D. Jr., Land, C.E., Shore, R.E., et al., Risk of breast cancer following low dose radiation exposure, Radiology, 131(3):589–597, 1979

4. Miller, A.B., Howe, G.R., Sherman, G.J., et al. Mortality from breast cancer after irradiation during fluoroscopic examinations in patients being treated for tuberculosis, New England Journal of Medicine, 321(19):1285–1289, 1989

5. U.S. Department of Health, Education and Welfare, Gonad Shielding in Diagnostic Radiology, DHEW Publication (FDA) 75-8024, Rockville, MD, June, 1975

6. Godderidge, C., Female gonadal shielding, Applied Radiology, 8(2):65–67, 1979

7. National Council on Radiation Protection and Measurements, Report No. 68, Radiation Protection in Pediatric Radiology, National Council on Radiation Protection and Measurements, Bethesda, MD, 1981

Chapter 15

Typical Radiation Exposures and Doses During Common Pediatric Examinations

Keith J. Strauss

INTRODUCTION

Table 15–1 lists typical pediatric patient exposures to radiation and resulting radiation doses as a function of patient size for specific plain radiographic examinations. The exposures and doses listed in Table 15–1 are defined and explained, parameters that affect the results of the measurements and calculations are discussed, the results of the data are summarized, and the trends are explained.

The typical data in Table 15–1 allow comparisons of exposures and doses relative to changes in patient size and in the type of plain radiographic examination. Actual exposures and doses to a patient can differ from these data by a factor of more than two. These data must not be used to calculate a specific patient's exposure and dose. Rather, a qualified radiologic physicist should periodically measure each machine's radiation output to verify that patient exposures and resultant doses are reasonable.

RADIATION EXPOSURE AND DOSE

X-rays (photons or electromagnetic waves) in nature transport energy from one location to another. As the x-ray beam passes through air (with its load of energy), some x-rays interact with the electrons in their shells of air molecules.[1] Electrons are separated (ionized) from their parent atom, producing positive and negative ions. The quantity of ions produced is dependent on the energy carried by all the photons. This is equal to the number of x-rays in the beam and the quantity of energy carried by each x-ray. If one counts the number of ions produced, one measures the exposure,[1] which is the quantity of energy (total amount of radiation) carried by an x-ray beam through air to a specific location in air, e.g., the entrance skin plane.

X-rays that reach the entrance skin plane of the patient travel through the patient's tissue in a straight line (unattenuated x-rays), change directions (scattered x-rays) and continue their travel, or stop (absorbed x-rays). The unattenuated x-rays that do not interact with the tissues and exit from the patient's body in a straight line are used to form the diagnostic image on film.[2] These x-rays have no effect on the patient's tissue.[3] If the x-ray changes direction or is stopped, some or all of its energy, respectively, must be transferred (unloaded) from the x-ray to the molecules of the tissue. Because scattering (change in direction) results in a partial unloading of the x-ray's energy to the tissue, the remaining energy continues to be carried by the scattered x-ray. When the x-ray is completely absorbed, all of its energy is transferred to the tissue and the x-ray ceases to exist. Dose[2] is the measure of the quantity of energy that is transferred (unloaded) to the tissue per mass of tissue at a specific location in the patient's body as the result of the scattering or absorption of an x-ray. This transferred energy does affect the patient's tissues. If the unloaded or deposited energy (dose) is sufficient, radiobiological damage occurs.

The interrelationships of exposure and dose can be explained using the analogy of a freight train carrying coal. The total quantity of coal on the train (total energy in the x-ray beam) is equal to the coal in each car (energy of each x-ray) times the number of cars (number of x-rays). If the train passes through a town without stopping, no coal was delivered; the town was "exposed" to the train but received no "dose" of coal. If the train stops in a town, unloads some of its coal, and then continues its journey, the town was exposed to the train and received a dose of coal. The dose that results from an exposure is dependent on actions taken to unload the train in the town. With x-rays, the amount of dose that results from a given exposure is determined by how the x-rays interact with the patient's tissues as the x-rays pass through a specific location in the tissue.

A typical dosimeter used to measure exposure uses an ionization chamber that counts the ions produced within the chamber's air volume. The familiar unit of exposure is the roentgen (R), but the International System (SI) unit is coulombs per kilogram.[4] The coulomb (C) is a unit of charge used to quantify the number of ions, while a kilogram (kg) is a measure of the mass of the air sample in which the charges were created. The conversion between the two systems of units is[2]

$$1 \text{ R} = 2.58 \times 10^{-4} \text{ C/kg} \tag{1}$$

$$1 \text{ C/kg} = 3876 \text{ R} \tag{2}$$

In either system, the quantity is defined in air only for photons with energy values less than 3 MeV[1]. One can properly discuss the entrance skin exposure of the patient, but exposures are not defined for the patient's internal organs because these organs are not "in air."

Patient doses to radiation are typically calculated with experimentally determined conversion data applied to measured exposure values. The familiar unit of dose is the rad. The SI unit is the Gray (Gy).[2]

$$1 \text{ rad} = 0.01 \text{ Gy} \tag{3}$$

$$1 \text{ Gy} = 100 \text{ rad} \tag{4}$$

The dose within the patient's body as a result of a uniform whole-body x-ray exposure is not uniform. Doses to tissues at shallow depths are significantly higher than doses to tissues at lower depths because the shallow tissues stop (absorb) the lower energy x-rays and prevent this energy from being delivered to the lower depths. Different organs of the body located at the same depth can receive significantly different doses owing to the molecular makeup and chemical structure of the different organs. For example, at diagnostic x-ray energies the rad/roentgen conversion factors for muscle and bone are approximately 0.95 and 3, respectively.[1] This means the dose to bone is approximately three times higher than the dose to soft tissues at the same depth. For these reasons, the term *patient dose* has little meaning. One needs to specify the dose to a specific organ (e.g., gonadal dose) or to a specific location in the patient's body (e.g., entrance, midline, exit).

Entrance skin doses are calculated from free-in-air exposure values determined for a specific machine. First, the dose in air is calculated at the skin entrance plane. However, the patient's tissue at shallow depths causes some of the x-rays to backscatter (reverse direction) after the x-rays pass by the skin. These backscattered x-rays elevate the skin dose. This is accounted for by applying a backscatter factor, which depends on the energy of the x-rays and the size of the x-ray beam.[1]

$$\text{Skin dose} = X \cdot f \cdot B \tag{5}$$

where X = the measured free-in-air exposure, f = the rad/roentgen conversion factor for air[1] ($\sim$0.9), and B = the backscatter factor[5] (1.03 − 1.15).

Midline doses are typically calculated. The midline dose underestimates the dose received by the tissues between the entrance plane and the midline of the patient and overestimates the dose received by tissue between the midline and the exit plane.

$$\text{Midline dose (D)} = D_s \cdot D/D_s \tag{6}$$

where D = the dose at midline, D_s = the skin dose, and D/D_s = the percent depth dose factor. Typical values of D/D_s[6] range from 0.99 to 0 depending on the thickness of the body part, the energy of the x-rays, the collimated x-ray field size, and the distance from the focal spot to the point of interest.

Specific *organ doses* of relatively radiosensitive organs (e.g., thyroid, gonads), which may or may not lie in the primary field of the x-ray beam during the radiographic examination, are an alternative to midline doses. Other doses (*integral dose*,[2] *effective dose*,[7] and *exposure area product* or *surface integral exposure*[2]) are sometimes calculated to assist with the assessment of radiation risk associated with a particular examination.

MEASUREMENT OF EXPOSURE AND CALCULATION OF DOSES

The determination of the free-in-air entrance exposure associated with a specific radiographic examination on a specific machine begins with the measurement of the radiation output (exposure) of the particular machine. The total energy emitted by the x-ray tube (exposure) during a specific examination depends on the rate (mA) at which the machine produces x-rays, how long the x-rays are produced (exposure time), and the energy each x-ray carries (selected high voltage [kVp]). The rate and energy of each x-ray are dependent on the following:

1. X-ray generator type (e.g., single phase, three phase, frequency inverter)
2. Target material of the anode (e.g., tungsten, molybdenum, rhodium)
3. Total filtration in the x-ray beam (millimeters of aluminum equivalence)
4. Distance from the source of the x-rays (focal spot)
5. Selected high voltage
6. Selected tube current (milliamperes [mA])

The above list assumes that the x-ray generator is calibrated (i.e., indicated radiographic technique factors and actual values are equal). If the machine is properly calibrated, the rate of exposure for a specific machine for a given radiographic technique should be independent of the selected focal spot size.

After the exposure rate is measured at a standard high voltage, tube current, and distance associated with a specific machine, one may calculate the free-in-air entrance exposure associated with a patient of a specific size and a specific radiographic examination if one knows the following additional items:

1. Selected high voltage for the examination (kVp)
2. Selected tube current for the examination (mA)
3. Selected exposure time (seconds [s]) for the examination
4. Distance from the source of the x-rays (focal spot) to the entrance plane of the patient (source-skin distance [SSD])

$$SSD = SID - PID - PT \qquad (7)$$

where SID = source-image distance, PID = patient exit plane to image receptor distance, and PT = patient thickness.

The appropriate values of kVp, mA, and s for a specific patient and specific machine are affected by the following:

1. SSD
2. Patient thickness

3. Patient composition, which can be dependent on the disease state (e.g., pneumonia)
4. Attenuating materials in the beam in front of the image receptor
   a. Tabletop thickness and composition (e.g., standard vs. carbon fiber)
   b. Automatic exposure control (AEC) device pickup (thickness and composition)
   c. Grid
       i. Presence or absence
      ii. Ratio (e.g., 6:1 vs. 12:1)
     iii. Lines per inch (e.g., 60 vs. 150 lines/inch)
      iv. Cover and interspace material (e.g., standard vs. carbon fiber)
       v. Focal range and alignment
   d. Cassette front thickness and composition (e.g. standard vs. carbon fiber)

5. Speed of image receptor
   a. Manufacturer's design
   b. Optimal film processing
       i. Film manufacturer's recommended chemistry
      ii. Optimal developer temperature
     iii. Recommended chemistry replenishment rates

Because the exposure at a point of interest (skin surface of a patient) from an x-ray source varies as $1/d^2$ where d = the distance between the source and the point of interest,[2] the SSD for a given clinical examination will affect the operator's choice of kVp, mA, and s to provide the proper number of x-rays at the image receptor.

For each half value layer (HVL) of thickness that the patient increases in size (~3.5 cm of tissue at 70 kVp)[4], the mAs value or quantity of x-rays required must double if the kVp is unchanged. For example, at 70 kVp, if the patient's abdomen increases from 18 to 21 cm in thickness, the chosen mAs must be doubled for the larger patient despite the fact that the thickness increased only 17% with respect to the original 18 cm. Any disease state of the patient that increases the density of the tissue (e.g., fluid-filled lung) increases the required number of x-rays.

The attenuating properties of all the materials between the patient and image receptor affect the number of x-rays that must be used at the entrance plane of the patient to deliver the correct number of x-rays to the image receptor. The high-quality, standard tabletop listed in the section on radiographic equipment attenuates approximately 18% of the primary x-rays at 80 kVp; a carbon fiber tabletop, depending on thickness, would reduce patient exposure 3% to 15%.[8]

Ideally, the AEC device pickup and the front cover of the cassette of the image receptor should not absorb any x-rays. The AEC pickup device listed in the section on radiographic equipment attenuates approximately 8% of the primary x-rays at 80 kVp. The attenuation of the front cover of the X-Omatic cassettes listed in the section on radiographic equipment is approximately 20% at 80 kVp. Carbon fiber cassette fronts would allow significant reduction in patient exposure.[8]

The type of grid used and its presence or absence significantly affect the patient dose during an examination. The presence of a grid as opposed to no grid increases patient exposure[4] by a factor of 2 to 4, depending on the size of the patient, the kVp used, and the size of the collimated x-ray field, all of which affect the amount of scattered x-rays generated. Most of the increase in exposure is required to compensate for the loss of density on the radiograph due to the elimination by the grid of most of the scattered x-rays. Because the scatter levels are low when thin body parts of pediatric patients are imaged with small x-ray fields at low kVp values, significant sparing of patient exposure and dose can be achieved by the removal of the grid without significant loss of radiographic contrast.

When a grid is necessary to maintain radiographic contrast by removing excessive scatter, the ideal grid should pass all unscattered x-rays and attenuate all scattered x-rays. However, the lead strips of the grid and the aluminum interspaces between the strips attenuate some of the unscattered x-rays, resulting in increased patient exposure and dose. This increase can be minimized by selecting a grid with a lead content just sufficient to remove most of the scattered x-rays and selecting a cover material such as carbon instead of aluminum. (The lead content in the grid is dependent on the grid ratio and the number of lines per inch in the grid.)[4] Studies have shown that carbon fiber interspace and cover materials compared with aluminum attenuate 20% to 30% fewer x-rays.[8] Grids attenuate 30% to 50% of the unscattered x-rays, depending on their lead content.[9]

Grid alignment and the grid's focal range are two parameters that can result in unnecessary patient exposure and dose. If the grid is upside down, tilted, or off-center with respect to the focal spot, the focused lead strips project a shadow that is greater than the strip width (grid cutoff). If the focal spot falls outside the focal range of the grid, the same problem occurs. These misalignment problems, depending on their severity, can easily increase attenuation of the unscattered x-rays by 30% to 40%,[4] which increases patient exposure and dose values by the same amount.

Image receptors are designed to have a unique speed that affects the patient dose. This speed is dependent on the fraction of the incident photons that interact with the fluorescent screens and the amount of light the screens generate with respect to the x-ray energy absorbed.[4] As the speed of an image receptor is increased, fewer x-rays are required at the image receptor to produce the proper density on the radiograph. The chosen speed of an image receptor should be determined by the amount of quantum mottle (noise) in the image that the radiologist can tolerate.

Film processing is too often overlooked by the operator; if faulty, it can cause a significant loss of image receptor speed. Typical quality control testing performed on the processor verifies that the processing is consistent from day to day, but it does not detect substandard processing that prevents the film from obtaining its designed speed. First, the speed of most films is degraded if the film manufacturer's recommended brand of chemistry (developer and fixer) is not used in the processor.[10] Second, the temperatures of the developer and the fixer in their respective tanks in the processor must be matched with the transport time of the processor according to the manufacturer's specifications. Finally, the rate at which replenishment chemicals (developer and fixer) are pumped into the developer and fixer tanks must be sufficient to replace the depleted chemicals and maintain the proper active ingredients over time.[10]

EXPOSURE AND DOSE TABLE

Table 15–1 lists typical free-in-air entrance exposure values (mR) and doses (mrad) from common plain radiographic examinations for patients ranging from newborns to adults. These data result from the use of state-of-the-art, quality x-ray equipment performing optimally (described below) and from the use of the radiographic techniques (kVp, mA, s) and distances listed in the table. The data provided allow comparisons of exposures and doses relative to changes in patient size and the type of plain radiographic examination. The exposure and dose for a specific patient is dependent on the radiographic technique used, the patient's unique anatomy and disease state, and the performance and setup of the specific x-ray equipment. Use of nonoptimal radiographic techniques or of nonoptimized equipment can easily result in exposure and dose values that differ from the typical values listed in the table by more than a factor of 2. Questions concerning exposure and dose for a specific patient should be answered by a qualified diagnostic radiologic physicist who periodically measures each machine's radiation output.

Text continued on p. 220

Table 15–1
TYPICAL RADIATION EXPOSURES AND DOSES

Patient Age	SID' (cm)	PID (cm)	Grd. Rat.	kVp	mAs	Pat. Thick. (cm)	Free A. Expos. (mR) ±10%	Skin ±15%	Doses (mrad) Midline ±30%	M/F° Gonads ±30%
POSTEROANTERIOR CHEST (400-SPEED)										
Adult	183	5	8	130	1.0	24	7.0	7.3	2.2	0.000/0.035
10–15 yr	183	5	—	85	2.4	19	7.5	7.5	2.3	—
6–10 yr	183	5	—	80	2.3	17	6.2	6.1	2.2	0.000/0.034
3–6 yr	183	2	—	75	2.1	14	4.9	4.8	2.1	0.000/0.008
1–3 yr	183	2	—	70	2.1	13	4.2	4.0	1.8	—
3–12 mo.	107	1	—	65	0.8	12	4.8	4.6	2.2	—
Newborn	107	1	—	60	0.8	10	3.9	3.6	2.1	0.012/0.047
LATERAL CHEST (400-SPEED)										
Adult	183	5	8	130	3.0	34	23	24	3.6	0.000/0.060
10–15 yr	183	5	—	100	2.4	28	11	11	2.0	—
6–10 yr	183	5	—	95	2.3	26	9.6	9.8	2.0	—
3–6 yr	183	2	—	90	2.1	19	7.3	7.4	2.4	0.000/0.073
1–3 yr	183	2	—	85	2.1	16	6.3	6.3	2.5	0.000/0.082
3–12 mo	107	1	—	70	0.8	13	5.7	5.5	2.5	—
Newborn	107	1	—	64	0.8	10	4.5	4.3	2.5	0.027/0.023
3-FOOT SPINE POSTEROANTERIOR (1100-SPEED)										
25–30 cm	183	4	10	85	30	27	103	103	17	1.9/31
20–25 cm	183	4	10	80	24	23	70	69	15	—
17–20 cm	183	4	10	75	20	18	49	48	15	—
13–17 cm	183	4	10	70	16	15	33	32	12	4.3/12
3-FOOT SPINE LATERAL (1100-SPEED)										
35–40 cm	183	4	10	95	60	32	272	277	35	2.0/30
30–35 cm	183	4	10	90	48	29	189	191	29	—
27–30 cm	183	4	10	85	40	25	135	135	26	—
23–27 cm	183	4	10	80	32	22	93	92	22	15/26

Table continued on following page

Table 15-1

TYPICAL RADIATION EXPOSURES AND DOSES (Continued)

Patient Age	SID (cm)	PID (cm)	Grd. Rat.	kVp	mAs	Pat. Thick. (cm)	Free A. Expos. (mR) ±10%	Doses (mrad) Skin ±15%	Doses (mrad) Midline ±30%	Doses (mrad) M/F° Gonads ±30%
ANTEROPOSTERIOR KUB (400-SPEED)										
Adult	107	8	8	85	5.0	21	63	63	15	1.6/18
10–15 yr	107	8	8	80	5.0	18	52	51	15	—
6–10 yr	107	8	8	75	3.8	16	33	32	11	—
3–6 yr	107	8	8	75	3.0	14	25	24	10	3.1/8.9
1–3 yr	107	8	8	70	3.0	13	21	20	8.6	2.2/7.4
3–12 mo	107	8	8	65	2.2	12	15	14	6.4	—
Newborn	107	8	8	65	1.5	10	8.6	8.2	4.5	1.2/4.8
ANTEROPOSTERIOR PELVIS AND HIPS (400-SPEED)										
Adult	107	8	8	85	4.0	22	51	51	11	5.1/14
10–15 yr	107	8	8	80	4.0	19	43	43	11	—
6–10 yr	107	8	8	80	2.0	17	20	20	6.4	—
3–6 yr	107	8	8	70	1.9	15	14	13	4.7	5.2/14
1–3 yr	107	8	8	70	1.5	14	12	12	4.5	4.4/12
3–12 mo	107	8	8	70	1.5	13	11	11	4.5	—
Newborn	107	8	8	65	1.3	11	7.6	7.2	3.6	4.3/7.6
ANTEROPOSTERIOR LUMBAR SPINE (400-SPEED)										
Adult	107	8	8	85	6.0	21	75	75	18	0.30/9.0
10–15 yr	107	8	8	80	5.2	18	54	53	16	—
6–10 yr	107	8	8	80	3.8	16	38	38	13	—
3–6 yr	107	8	8	75	3.0	14	25	24	9.9	2.8/6.3
1–3 yr	107	8	8	70	2.2	13	16	15	6.5	1.7/5.1
3–12 mo	107	8	8	70	2.0	12	14	13	6.2	—
Newborn	107	8	8	70	1.5	10	10	10	5.5	1.1/4.3
LUMBAR SPINE LATERAL (400-SPEED)										
Adult	107	8	8	95	12.0	28	222	226	33	0.29/15
10–15 yr	107	8	8	90	10.0	24	150	152	29	—
6–10 yr	107	8	8	85	7.6	22	98	98	21	—
3–6 yr	107	8	8	85	6.0	18	70	70	21	9.1/16
1–3 yr	107	8	8	80	3.2	16	32	32	11	6.4/14
3–12 mo	107	8	8	75	3.0	13	24	23	10	—
Newborn	107	8	8	75	1.5	10	11	11	6.3	3.3/4.7

ANTEROPOSTERIOR OR LATERAL ELBOW (100-SPEED)

Age										
Adult	107	—	—	76	1.8	9	14	14	8.8	0.000/0.000
10–15 yr	107	—	—	74	1.3	8	9.2	8.9	6.2	—
6–10 yr	107	—	—	72	1.1	7	7.2	6.9	5.2	
3–6 yr	107	—	—	68	0.9	6	5.2	5.0	4.1	0.000/0.000
1–3 yr	107	—	—	66	0.9	4	4.7	4.5	3.9	0.000/0.000
3–12 mo	107	—	—	64	0.9	3	4.3	4.1	3.7	—
Newborn	107	—	—	62	0.9	2	3.9	3.7	3.4	0.000/0.000

ANTEROPOSTERIOR HAND (100-SPEED)

Age										
Adult	107	—	—	68	1.0	4.5	5.6	5.4	3.6	0.000/0.000
10–15 yr	107	—	—	68	0.8	3.5	4.4	4.2	3.0	—
6–10 yr	107	—	—	66	0.7	2.5	3.5	3.3	2.6	
3–6 yr	107	—	—	64	0.7	2.5	3.3	3.1	2.6	0.000/0.000
1–3 yr	107	—	—	62	0.7	2.0	3.1	2.9	2.5	0.000/0.000
3–12 mo	107	—	—	60	0.7	1.5	2.8	2.6	2.2	—
Newborn	107	—	—	58	0.6	1.0	2.2	2.0	1.9	0.000/0.000

ANTEROPOSTERIOR OR LATERAL KNEE (100-SPEED)

Age										
Adult	107	—	—	75	2.5	12	20	19	9.5	—
10–15 yr	107	—	—	75	2.1	11	16	16	8.4	—
6–10 yr	107	—	—	72	1.5	9	10	10	6.1	—
3–6 yr	107	—	—	72	0.7	7	4.6	4.4	3.3	—
1–3 yr	107	—	—	70	0.7	6	4.3	4.0	3.2	—
3–12 mo	107	—	—	66	0.7	4	3.6	3.4	3.0	—
Newborn	107	—	—	62	0.7	3	3.1	2.9	2.7	—

ANTEROPOSTERIOR FOOT (100-SPEED)

Age										
Adult	107	—	—	72	1.4	8	9.4	9.0	6.2	—
10–15 yr	107	—	—	72	0.8	7	5.3	5.1	3.8	—
6–10 yr	107	—	—	70	0.8	6	4.8	4.6	3.8	—
3–6 yr	107	—	—	68	0.8	5	4.5	4.3	3.7	—
1–3 yr	107	—	—	66	0.8	4	4.2	4.0	3.5	—
3–12 mo	107	—	—	64	0.6	3	2.9	2.8	2.5	—
Newborn	107	—	—	62	0.6	2	2.6	2.4	2.3	—

Table continued on following page

Table 15–1
TYPICAL RADIATION EXPOSURES AND DOSES (Continued)

Patient Age	SID* (cm)	PID (cm)	Grd. Rat.	kVp	mAs	Pat. Thick. (cm)	Free A. Expos. (mR) ±10%	Skin ±15%	Doses (mrad)	
									Midline ±30%	M/F° Gonads ±30%
ANTEROPOSTERIOR SKULL (400-SPEED)										
Adult	107	8	8	75	11.0	20	105	102	24	0.000/0.000
10–15 yr	107	8	8	75	9.0	18	83	81	23	—
6–10 yr	107	8	8	75	7.4	16	65	63	21	—
3–6 yr	107	8	8	75	5.6	15	48	47	17	0.000/0.000
1–3 yr	107	8	8	70	3.7	14	27	26	10	0.000/0.000
3–12 mo	107	8	8	70	2.9	13	21	20	8.6	—
Newborn	107	8	8	70	2.3	12	16	15	7.1	0.000/0.000
AXIAL SKULL (400-SPEED)										
Adult	107	8	8	85	11.0	22	141	141	31	0.000/0.000
10–15 yr	107	8	8	85	9.0	21	111	111	26	—
6–10 yr	107	8	8	85	7.4	18	86	86	26	—
3–6 yr	107	8	8	85	5.6	17	63	63	21	0.000/0.000
1–3 yr	107	8	8	80	3.7	16	37	37	13	0.000/0.000
3–12 mo	107	8	8	80	2.9	15	28	28	11	—
Newborn	107	8	8	80	2.3	14	22	22	9.2	0.000/0.000
LATERAL SKULL (400-SPEED)										
Adult	107	8	8	70	11.0	18	87	84	22	0.000/0.000
10–15 yr	107	8	8	70	9.0	16	69	66	21	—
6–10 yr	107	8	8	70	7.4	15	55	53	19	—
3–6 yr	107	8	8	70	5.6	14	41	39	15	0.000/0.000
1–3 yr	107	8	8	65	3.7	12	22	20	9.4	0.000/0.000
3–12 mo	107	8	8	65	2.9	11	17	16	8.1	—
Newborn	107	8	8	65	2.3	10	13	12	6.9	0.000/0.000

POSTEROANTERIOR AXIAL SINUSES (400-SPEED)

Adult	115	4	8	85	6.9	22	84	84	19	0.000/0.000
10–15 yr	115	4	8	85	6.6	21	78	78	19	—
6–10 yr	115	4	8	80	6.2	18	61	60	19	0.000/0.000
3–6 yr	115	4	8	80	5.9	17	57	56	19	0.000/0.000
1–3 yr	115	4	8	75	5.5	16	46	45	15	—
3–12 mo	115	4	8	70	3.7	15	26	25	9.0	—

WATERS METHOD SINUSES (400-SPEED)

Adult	115	4	8	90	6.9	22	93	94	22	0.000/0.000
10–15 yr	115	4	8	90	6.6	21	86	87	22	—
6–10 yr	115	4	8	85	6.2	18	69	69	22	0.000/0.000
3–6 yr	115	4	8	85	5.9	17	64	64	22	0.000/0.000
1–3 yr	115	4	8	80	5.5	16	52	51	18	—
3–12 mo	115	4	8	75	3.7	15	30	29	11	—

LATERAL SINUSES (400-SPEED)

Adult	115	4	8	70	8.0	18	52	50	14	0.000/0.000
10–15 yr	115	4	8	70	7.6	16	48	46	15	—
6–10 yr	115	4	8	70	7.2	15	44	42	15	0.000/0.000
3–6 yr	115	4	8	70	6.8	14	41	39	16	0.000/0.000
1–3 yr	115	4	8	60	6.4	12	27	25	11	—
3–12 mo	115	4	8	60	4.3	11	18	17	8.3	—

*SID = source-image distance. PID = patient exit plane to image receptor. Grd. Rat. = grid ratio. Pat. Thick. = patient thickness. Free A. Expos. = free-in-air exposure without scatter.
M/F = male/female.
†No gonadal shielding used.

RADIOGRAPHIC EQUIPMENT

Appendix D outlines the equipment used to collect the data presented in Table 15–1. These data are provided for radiographers who, with the assistance of their radiologic physicist, wish to evaluate their institution's patient radiation exposures and doses with respect to these results. The following paragraph summarizes the nonstandard features of the equipment used.

All grid ratios are less than 12:1, the typical value used for adults. The selected 8:1 and 10:1 grids provide adequate lead content to remove the lower levels of scattered x-rays present during pediatric examinations, with some savings in patient exposure and dose due to less attenuation of the unscattered x-rays. The equipment used for sinus examinations has a fixed SID of 115 cm. The general equipment has an SID of 107 cm, selected to ensure adequate coverage of a 17-inch image receptor with an x-ray tube anode of only 12 degrees. X-ray tubes with 12-degree anode angles were chosen to improve the loadability of the anode with small nominal focal spots of 0.3 to 0.6 mm. The wall Buckys have two interchangeable grids—one focused at 72 inches and one focused at 40 inches to avoid the grid cutoff at SID values of either 40 or 72 inches that would result from a single grid. Because the 36-inch cassettes are used primarily for scoliosis examinations, in which radiologists can tolerate elevated levels of quantum mottle during interpretation, 1100-speed image receptors were selected for these large cassettes to reduce patient exposure.

DESCRIPTION OF THE DATA IN THE EXPOSURE AND DOSE TABLE

The data in Table 15–1 are grouped by specific examination. The image receptor speed used is listed in parentheses immediately after the label of the examination.

Column 1 lists patient age from newborn to adult.

Column 2 is the distance from the focal spot to the image receptor (SID). For a given examination, the SID remains constant except for posteroanterior and lateral chest radiographs. Only patients younger than 1 year are positioned supine on the tabletop, with an SID of 107 cm; all other chest radiographs are obtained with the patient upright, with an SID of 183 cm.

Column 3 is the distance from the exit plane of the patient to the image receptor (PID), which is determined by the device used to hold the image receptor (table Bucky, 8 cm; wall Bucky, 5 cm; 36-inch wall cassette holder 4 cm; upright cassette holder on table, 2 cm; tabletop exposures, 1 cm).

Column 4 lists the grid ratio. If no grid is used, a dash is entered.

Column 5 and 6, respectively, list the selected kVp and mAs used during the examination. The kVp is selected based on desired radiographic contrast. The mAs is selected to obtain the proper radiographic density at the selected kVp.

Column 7 lists the average thickness of the body part radiographed for the patient age listed in the first column.

Columns 8 through 11 contain data that were calculated.

Column 8 lists the free-in-air entrance exposure in mR that results from the use of the indicated kVp and mAs at the clinical SSD (equation 7). For a given machine, each entry in column 8 could be measured directly. In this case, a computer program developed by Nuclear Associates, called Radcomp, was used to calculate these exposures. The measured half-value layer (HVL) at a known kVp and five measured exposure values in mR/mAs at 50, 70, 90, 110, and 130 kVp on the x-ray machine in question are entered into the computer program. From these data the program calculates the free-in-air exposure values at the SSD for each requested clinical kVp, mAs, and patient thickness.[11] Each calculated value in column 8 should be accurate to ±10%.

Column 9 lists the entrance skin dose (in millirads) that is associated with each entrance skin exposure listed in column 8. This is calculated using equation 5. The rad/roentgen conversion factor[1] and backscatter factors[5] were taken from experimental data. The calculated values in column 9 should be accurate to ±15%.

Column 10 lists the midline dose (in millirads) associated with the entrance skin exposures listed in column 8. Theoretically, these values could be calculated from the values in column 9 using equation 6. However, direct percent depth dose factors for the varying SSD values associated with pediatric patients are not readily available. Therefore, the midline doses were calculated from the free-in-air entrance exposure values in column 8 using the appropriate rad/roentgen conversion factors,[1] tissue-air ratios,[5] and inverse square law corrections.[1] The values in column 10 should be accurate for the typical patient to within ±30%. The possible error is large because the tissue-air ratios and rad/roentgen conversion factors were experimentally determined for water. Although water is a reasonable model of homogeneous soft tissue, the presence of other materials (e.g., air, bone) can significantly alter the actual midline dose.

Column 11 lists the male/female gonadal doses associated with the entrance exposure values listed in column 8. These doses were calculated from the free-in-air entrance exposure values in column 8 using available rad/roentgen conversion factors for gonadal doses.[12] The selected conversion factors assumed that no gonadal shielding was used and that for pediatric examinations, the x-ray field was collimated to the size of the body part examined rather than to the size of the image receptor. If the calculated value was <0.001 mrad, the value listed in the table is 0.000 mrad. Values are listed only for adults, age ranges 3–6 and 1–3, and newborns; rad/roentgen conversion factors were available for only these age groups.[12] The values in column 11 should be accurate for the typical patient to within ±30%. The assumed errors are large because the rad/roentgen conversion factors were experimentally determined with specific collimated x-ray field sizes or SID values that were not always identical to the collimated x-ray field sizes or SID values used in Table 15–1.

VARIANCES IN THE DATA

The listed accuracies of the various calculated values (±10% to 30%) are small compared with the variation in the calculated values, which can result from nonoptimized equipment, different choices of radiographic technique, or typical variances in patient anatomy. Large variations in patient tissue density occur for the same size patient, depending on body build. Measured entrance exposure values on patients[13,14] have shown variations of a factor of 2 or more for patients of the same size.

Choice of kVp also significantly affects the entrance exposure value. Assume that the chosen kVp for an anteroposterior radiograph of the kidney, ureter, and bladder (KUB) of a child 1 to 3 years old is changed ±10 kVp with respect to the 70 kVp used in Table 15–1. The first, second, and third rows, respectively, of the data in Table 15–2 is the case of −10 kVp, original kVp, and +10 kVp.

One notes that the entrance exposure is 43% greater at 60 kVp than at 70 kVp and 24% less at 80 kVp than at 70 kVp. The midline dose is 28% greater at 60 kVp than at 70 kVp and 14% less at 80 kVp than at 70 kVp. As one would expect, as the kVp increases, the gonadal doses for the same examination decrease significantly. Clearly, the changes in the calculated example of a simple choice of radiographic technique can be significant.

Table 15-2
CHANGES IN RADIATION EXPOSURES AND DOSES AS kVp CHANGES

Patient Age	SID* (cm)	PID (cm)	Grd. Rat.	kVp	mAs	Pat. Thick. (cm)	Free A. Expos. (mR) ±10%	Skin ±15%	Midline ±30%	M/F Gonads ±30%
								Doses (mrad)		
ANTEROPOSTERIOR KUB (400-SPEED)										
1–3 yr	107	8	8	60	5.8	13	30	28	11	3.2/11
1–3 yr	107	8	8	70	3.0	13	21	20	8.6	2.2/7.8
1–3 yr	107	8	8	80	1.8	13	16	16	7.3	1.7/6.4

*SID = source-image distance, PID = patient exit plane to image receptor, Grd. Rat. = grid ratio, Pat. Thick. = patient thickness, Free A. Expos. = free-in-air exposure without scatter, M/F = male/female.

For these reasons, the data in Table 15–1 are provided only to allow *comparisons* of exposures and doses *relative* to changes in patient size and the type of plain radiographic examination. The data should not be used to estimate the free-in-air exposure and dose values for a specific patient examined on a specific machine unless a diagnostic radiologic physicist has verified by direct measurement of the machine's radiation output that the data in the tables are appropriate for the specific machine and its setup.

SUMMARY OF THE RESULTS

The calculated values in Table 15–1, free-in-air exposure, skin dose, midline dose, and the male/female gonadal doses vary as a function of patient age.

FREE-IN-AIR EXPOSURE

The increase in free-in-air exposure (column 8) relative to patient thickness is dependent on the selected range of kVp and the density of the tissue under examination. For chest examinations (low density and 60 to 130 kVp):

$$X \; \alpha \; t \tag{8}$$

where X = free-in-air entrance exposure, α = is proportional to, and t = thickness of the patient. As chest thickness doubles, free-in-air entrance exposure doubles.

For relatively dense body parts imaged over a smaller range of kVp <20, (e.g., 3-foot spine 40-inch spine, KUB, pelvis and hip, and sinus examinations):

$$X \; \alpha \; t^3 \tag{9}$$

As abdomen thickness doubles, free-in-air entrance exposure increases by a factor of 8.

For skull examinations, a relatively dense body part with no change in kVp:

$$X \; \alpha \; t^4 \tag{10}$$

ENTRANCE SKIN DOSE

The skin dose values (column 9) relative to the free-in-air entrance exposures range from 4% greater at 130 kVp to 7% less at 60 kVp. At 85 kVp the skin dose is identical to the free-in-air entrance exposure values. Because these dose values are similar in all cases to the free-in-air entrance exposures, the skin dose values as a function of patient thickness are the same as described in the previous paragraph.

MIDLINE DOSE

For all body parts with any significant thickness > 10 cm, the change in midline dose as a function of patient size (column 10) is less than the change in either free-in-air entrance exposure values or skin doses. Equation 6 explains this result. The percent depth dose factor in equation 6 decreases as patient thickness increases because more attenuating tissue lies between the entrance and midline planes. At the same time, free-in-air exposure values increase with patient thickness. The increasing and decreasing factors in the same equation offset each other.

For the posteroanterior chest examination (wide range of kVp), the midline dose is constant as a function of changing thickness. For the lateral chest examination (larger variation in patient thickness), the midline dose increases only 50% from the newborn to the adult. For the denser body parts with a small change of kVp ≤ 20, (e.g., KUB, spine, and skull examinations), the midline dose triples as the entrance skin dose increases by a factor of 8. When the kVp is essentially unchanged (sinuses), the midline dose doubles as the skin dose triples.

Midline doses are considered to be better indicators of radiobiological risks than entrance doses.[3] Because entrance skin doses increase more rapidly than midline doses as a function of patient thickness, the use of entrance skin doses tends to overestimate radiobiological risks. This is particularly true in cases where the kVp increases significantly as a function of patient size (chest examination).

GONADAL DOSES

The gonadal doses that occur without shielding (column 11) range from undetectable to significant values. These values are dependent on the free-in-air entrance skin exposure and the proximity of the gonads to the primary x-ray beam. If the gonads are as little as 10 cm from the edge of the primary beam, the gonadal dose will be as little as 1% to 2% of the entrance dose.[12]

These values can be reduced by appropriate shielding in most cases. Shielding of the male gonads when in the primary beam can reduce doses to 10% to 20% of the values listed in Table 15–1.[12] These reduction factors will not be as low for shielded female gonads because the shield cannot be placed adjacent to the gonads. Gonadal dose reduction by shielding is much less significant for both male and female when the gonads are outside the primary beam; the external shielding is not effective at stopping scattered x-rays inside the patient from reaching the gonads. These internal scattered x-rays are the primary source of radiation dose to the gonads when the gonads are outside the primary beam.

Gonadal doses per radiograph that are smaller than the daily radiation dose from background radiation are considered insignificant in this discussion. The daily dose to the male gonads from background radiation at sea level is 0.25 mrad.[15] Owing to attenuation provided by overlying tissues, the corresponding daily dose to the female gonads is somewhat less. Therefore, gonadal doses associated with all examinations of the extremities and skull are clearly insignificant. The calculated gonadal doses associated with these examinations are all <0.001 mrad — at least 250 times less than the criteria level of 0.25 mrad. Whereas the gonadal doses associated with chest examinations are >0.001 mrad, these examinations deliver insignificant gonadal doses.

The gonadal doses associated with examinations of the abdomen, spine, and pelvis are significant when gonadal shielding is not used. For all these examinations the female gonads typically lie within the primary x-ray beam. This results in female gonadal doses that are approximately equal to the midline doses listed in column 10. For the male, the gonadal doses are determined by the proximity of the male gonads to the primary beam. With spine and abdomen examinations, the male gonadal dose is less than the midline dose. For anteroposterior hip examinations, the male gonads lie in the primary x-ray beam between the entrance and midline planes; the gonadal dose is greater than the midline dose.

In 1965 Aspin[16] published an extensive table of experimentally measured gonadal doses from diagnostic x-ray examinations, which has been adapted and republished by others.[17] The gonadal dose values listed in Table 15–1 are significantly less than those previously published for a number of reasons. In 1965, state-of-the-art x-ray wave forms resulted in greater patient doses[6] than state-of-the-art x-ray wave forms available today. Image receptors (screen/film combinations) were significantly slower in 1965 than today, and selected kVp values were lower.

REFERENCES

1. Johns, H.E., and Cunningham, J.R., The Physics of Radiology, Charles C Thomas, Springfield, IL., 1969
2. Sprawls, P. Jr., Physical Principles of Medical Imaging, Aspen Publishers, Rockville, MD, 1987.
3. Hall, E.J., Radiobiology for the Radiologist, Harper & Row, Hagerstown, MD, 1978
4. Curry, T.S. III, Dowdey, J.E., and Murry, R.C. Jr., Christensen's Introduction to the Physics of Diagnostic Radiology, Lea & Febiger, Philadelphia, 1990
5. Schulz, R.J., and Gignac, C.E., Applications of tissue-air ratio for patient dosage in diagnostic radiology, Radiology, 120:687–690, 1976
6. Kelley, J.P., and Trout, E.D., Physical characteristics of the radiation from 2 pulse, 12-pulse and 10000-pulse x-ray equipment, Radiology, 100:653–661, 1971
7. Huda, W., and Bissessur, K., Effective dose equivalents, H_E in diagnostic radiology, Medical Physics, 17(6):998–103, 1990
8. Hutton, A.P., and Russell, J.G., The use of carbon fibre material in table tops, cassette fronts, and grid covers, Magnitude of possible dose reduction, British Journal of Radiology, 59:157–163, 1986
9. Hondius, B.W., Grids to Reduce Scattered X-ray in Medical Radiography, Philips Research Reports Supplement No. 1, Philips Medical Systems, Inc., Eindhoven, Netherlands, 1964
10. Haus, A.G., Automatic film processing in medical imaging: System design considerations, in Specification, Acceptance Testing and Quality Control of Diagnostic X-ray Imaging Equipment, Proceedings of 1991 AAPM Summer School, Santa Cruz, CA, pp. 420–446, 1991
11. Zamenhof, R.G., Shahabi, S., and Morgan, H.T., An improved method for estimating the entrance exposure in diagnostic radiologic examinations, American Journal of Roentgenology, 149:631–637, 1987
12. Kereiakes, J.G., and Rosenstein, M., Handbook of Radiation Doses in Nuclear Medicine and Diagnostic X-ray, CRC Press, Boca Raton, FL, p. 252, 1980
13. Conway, B.J., Butler, P.F., Duff, J.E., et al. Beam quality independent attenuation phantom for estimating patient exposure from x-ray automatic exposure controlled chest examinations, Medical Physics, 11(6):827–832, 1984
14. Conway, B.J., Duff, J.E., Fewell, T.R., et al., A patient equivalent attenuation phantom for estimating patient exposures from automatic exposure controlled x-ray examinations of the abdomen and lumbosacral spine, Medical Physics, 17(3):448–453, 1990
15. Hall, E.J., Radiation and Life, Pergamon Press, New York, 1976
16. Aspin, N., The gonadal x-ray dose to children from diagnostic radiographic techniques, Radiology, 85:944–951, 1965
17. Kirks, D.R., Practical Pediatric Imaging: Diagnostic Radiology of Infants and Children, Boston, Little, Brown, & Company, 1991

Illustrated Handouts for Children*

*Courtesy of the Department of Radiology, Children's Hospital, Boston, Massachusetts

BARIUM ENEMA

THE CHILDREN'S HOSPITAL
MEDICAL CENTER

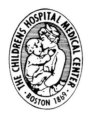

DEPARTMENT
OF
RADIOLOGY

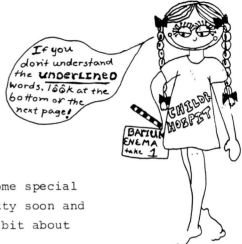

If you don't understand the **UNDERLINED** *words, look at the bottom of the next page!*

We heard you are going to have some special x-rays called a barium enema done pretty soon and we thought we would tell you a little bit about them so you'll know what's going on.

The barium enema is done in the <u>Radiology Department</u> of Children's Hospital. In this test the doctor will take some pictures of the lower part of your <u>digestive system</u> called the <u>colon</u>. You will miss breakfast if you have this test done in the morning; if you have it done in the afternoon, you will miss both breakfast and lunch. As soon as the test is over, you can eat again.

After you have gone to the bathroom, the <u>technologist</u> will ask you to take off your underpants and bring you into a large room where you'll see two big machines near a high metal table. These machines are just overgrown cameras which are hooked up to the two TV screens where you and your doctor can watch your insides. You will also see a plastic bag full of white liquid stuff called <u>barium</u> hung on a pole at one end of the table; a tube will be connected to this bag.

The doctor will ask you to get up on the table and lie on your left side with your knees pulled up close to your stomach. Then he will very gently slide the tube from the barium bag into your <u>anus</u>. But don't worry--he will make it very slippery so it will feel just like a thermometer. If you relax as much as you can, you won't feel much at all! The doctor will let some of the barium slowly run down the tube and into your colon. As he watches the TV screen, the doctor will stop and start the flow of barium. To get a better view of your colon, he may

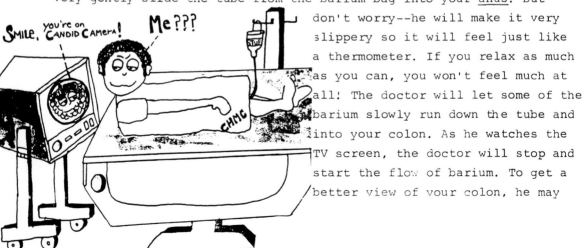

Smile, you're on CANDID CAMERA!

Me???

push on your stomach with a big black glove. He might also ask you to roll over on your sides or stomach so that he can photograph your best side. After a while you will begin to feel very full like when you really have to go to the bathroom on a car trip and there aren't any gas stations around. You'll feel better if you take long, deep breaths through your mouth.

When the TV screens flash on, the lights will go off and you will hear a low humming noise from the machine above you. When the doctor wants to take a picture, everything will happen in reverse--the lights will go on, the TV screens off, and for just a second there will be a loud noise like a train going by. For this second while the doctor takes a picture, you must lie very still so that the film will not come out blurry.

After the doctor has taken all the pictures he wants, the technologist will lead you into the room next door for just a couple more. Then you can go to the bathroom (finally!). After you have sat down for a few minutes, the technologist will take a few more pictures (this time minus the barium!), and then you're done. All you have to do is wait outside for a couple of minutes while your films are being developed. This is real service since your parents have to wait several weeks to have their photographs developed.

Radiology Department--the place in the hospital where x-rays are taken.

Digestive system--the part of you that is in charge of eating your food and grinding it up so that the rest of your body can use it. The colon comes at the bottom of your digestive system. It is where you store your bowel movements in between the times you go to the bathroom.

Technologist--the friendly person dressed in white who helps the doctors and answers any questions you have.

Barium--the white stuff that shows up very well on TV as it outlines the inside of your colon and makes it stand out.

Anus--the hole in your behind.

DJS & EAH
9/75

BARIUM SWALLOW AND UPPER GASTROINTESTINAL TRACT

Children's Hospital

**DEPARTMENT
OF
RADIOLOGY**

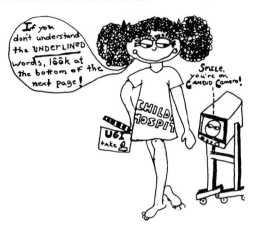

We heard you're going to have some special x-rays called a UGI done pretty soon and we thought we would tell you about them so you'll know what's going on.

The UGI is done in the <u>Radiology Department</u> of Children's Hospital. In this test, the doctor will take some pictures of your <u>digestive system</u>. You will miss breakfast if you have this test done in the morning; if you have it done in the afternoon, you will miss both breakfast and lunch. As soon as the test is over, you can eat again.

A <u>technologist</u> will bring you into a large room where you'll see two big machines near a high metal table. These machines are just overgrown cameras which are hooked up to two TV screens where you and your doctor can watch your stomach. The UGI will begin with you either standing up against the table or lying down on it, depending on the way the doctor likes to do things. Then the doctor will hand you a paper cup of <u>barium</u>. Try to swallow it exactly when the doctor tells you to. Sometimes the doctor will push your stomach in with a big black glove to move anything away that might be blocking his/her view. Also, he/she will ask you to think of your favorite foods so that your stomach will get excited and start working. If you started the test standing up,

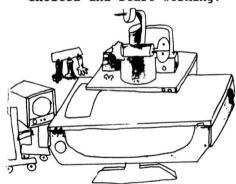

the doctor will give you a great ride on the table until you are lying down. If you want a ride but don't get one, just ask at the end of the test--they're pretty good about table rides. While you're lying down, the doctor will ask you to drink some more barium through a straw and tell you to turn over so that he can photograph your best side. (S)he will probably push your stomach some more.

When the TV screen flash on, the lights will go off and you will hear a low humming noise from the machine above you. After a few minutes, the doctor will want to take a picture; then everything will happen in reverse--the lights will go on, the TV screens off, and for just a second while the doctor takes a picture, you must lie very still so that the film will not come out blurry.

The swallows and the pictures are the only things that will happen in this test. Sometimes the doctor will ask you to go outside and drink some more barium. Then the technologist will take you into the room next door for some more pictures. After she/he has taken all the films the doctor wants, you'll be done! Then all you will have to do is wait outside for a few minutes while your pictures are being developed. This is real service since your parents have to wait several weeks to have their photographs developed.

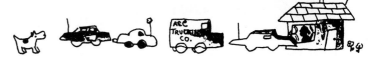

Radiology Department -- the place in the hospital where x-rays are taken.

Digestive system -- the part of you that is in charge of eating your food and grinding it up so that the rest of your body can use it. You will be able to see most of your digestive system on the TV screen during this test; just ask the doctor he/she will explain it to you.

Technologist -- the friendly person dressed in white who helps the doctor and answers any questions you have.

Spot film -- a quick picture of your chest and stomach that the doctor takes so he can zero in on the part of you he/she wants to look at.

Barium -- the pink stuff that looks like a strawberry milkshake and taste kind of chalky, but not too bad. If you look on the TV screen right after you swallow the barium, it will look black as it moves down the same path that your food follows. It is called contrast material because it makes your digestive system stand out from all of the other stuff in your body.

VOIDING CYSTOURETHROGRAM (BOYS)

Children's Hospital

DEPARTMENT
OF
RADIOLOGY

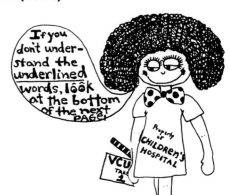

If you don't under- stand the underlined words, look at the bottom of the next page!

Property of CHILDREN'S HOSPITAL

VCU Test

We heard you are going to have some special x-rays called a VCUG done pretty soon and we thought we would tell you a little bit about them so you'll know what's going on. This test is done early in the morning in the <u>Radiology Department</u> of Children's Hospital. In the VCUG the doctor will take some pictures of your <u>bladder</u>.

After you have gone to the bathroom, the <u>technologist</u> will bring you into a large room where you will see a big machine over a high metal table. This machine is just an overgrown camera which is hooked up to a TV screen where you, your parents and your doctor can watch your bladder. You will also see a bottle full of clear liquid called <u>contrast material</u> hung on a pole at the end of the table; a thin plastic tube called a <u>catheter</u> will be connected to this bottle.

First the technologist will ask you to climb up on the table, lie down on your back, and slide off you underpants. The doctor will put on rubber gloves to keep you as clean as he can. Then he will wash off your penis very carefully with several pieces of cotton dipped in warm, pink colored soap. This is to make the area super clean, so you must be sure not to touch it until the test is over. Then the doctor or technologist will wash the soap off with warm water.

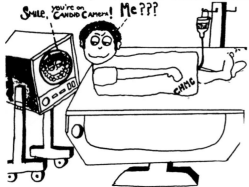

SMILE, you're on CANDID CAMERA! Me???

Then the doctor will put a very clean small blue cloth over you. The doctor will be touching your penis and this may feel a little funny, but this test is a real quickie and the more you relax the easier it will be. Then he might squirt some stuff into your penis with a kind of water pistol so that you will not feel anything. After a few minutes he will gently slide the catheter a little ways into your penis and loosely tape it to you so it doesn't come out during the test. Then the doctor will slowly let the liquid from the bottle run through the catheter and into your bladder. You will be able to watch your bladder fill up on the TV screen. As your bladder is filling, you will feel like you have to go to the bathroom. When you don't think that you can hold another drop, tell the doctor. He will tell you to hold it for just a few more seconds while he takes a couple of pictures. Then the technologist will give you a container to go to the bathroom in while you are still lying on the table; as you are going the plastic tube will slide out and the doctor will take some more pictures. When a picture is being taken you must lie very still so that the film does not come out blurry.

After the doctor has taken all of the pictures he or she wants, you're done! The technologist will wipe off any contrast material that has spilled on you during the test so you can put on your underpants and go outside to wait for a few minutes while your pictures are being developed. This is a real service since your parents have to wait several weeks to have their photographs developed.

P.S.   If it stings the next couple of times you go to the bathroom, don't worry, it will go away soon.

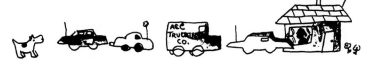

<u>Radiology Department</u> -- the place in the hospital where x-rays are taken.
<u>Bladder</u> -- the sac where you store your urine in between the times you go to the bathroom.
<u>Technologist</u> -- the very friendly person dressed in white pants or lab coat who helps the doctor and answers any questions you have.
<u>Contrast material</u> -- the liquid that the doctor puts into your bladder to make it look very round and dark on the TV screen so that he can see it more clearly.
<u>Catheter</u> -- if you haven't already guessed, this is the thin, slippery rubber tube that the doctor uses to get the contrast material from the bottle into your bladder.

VOIDING CYSTOURETHROGRAM (GIRLS)

Children's Hospital

**DEPARTMENT
OF
RADIOLOGY**

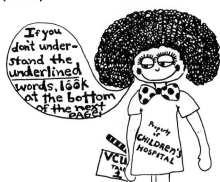

We heard you are going to have some special x-rays called a VCUG done pretty soon and we thought we would tell you a little bit about them so you'll know what's going on. This test is done in the morning in the <u>Radiology Department</u> of Children's Hospital. During the VCUG there will be some pictures taken of your <u>bladder</u>.

After you have gone to the bathroom, the <u>technologist</u> will bring you into a large room where you will see a big machine over a high metal table. This machine is just an overgrown camera which is hooked up to a TV screen where you and your doctor, and parents can watch your bladder. You will also see a bottle full of clear liquid called <u>contrast material</u> hung on a pole at the end of the table; a thin plastic tube called a <u>catheter</u> will be connected to this bottle.

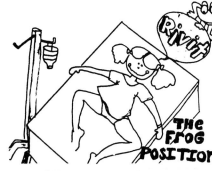

First the technologist will ask you to climb up on the table and lie on your back. The technologist will help you slide off your panties and ask you to pull your feet up close to your body sticking you knees out to the side like a frog. Then after putting on rubber gloves he or she will wash the area between your legs with some warm pink colored soap from a metal bowl, making you super clean, so until the end of the test you shouldn't touch anything below your belly-button. Then the doctor or technologist will wash off the soap with warm water and will put a very clean small blue cloth over you. Then he or she will gently slide the catheter a little ways into your <u>urethra</u> and the tube will be loosely taped to your leg so it won't fall out. After a little urine has been collected in a small cup, the stuff in the bottle will flow through the tube and into your bladder. You will be able to watch your bladder fill up on the TV screen. As your bladder is filling, you will feel like you have to go the bathroom. When you don't think you can hold another drop, tell the technologist and doctor. They will tell you to hold it for just a few more seconds while they take a couple of pictures. Then, believe it or not, they will ask you to go to the bathroom right on the table! While you are urinating they will be taking some more pictures of your bladder emptying.

When a picture is being taken, you must lie very still so that the film doesn't come out blurry.

After all of the pictures have been taken, you're done! The technologist will wipe off any contrast material that has spilled on you during the test so you can put your panties back on and go outside to wait for a few minutes while your pictures are being developed. This is real service since your parents have to wait for several days to have their photographs developed.

P.S.   If it stings the next couple of times you go to the bathroom, don't worry, it will go away soon.

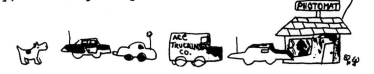

Radiology Department -- the place in the hospital where x-rays are taken.

Bladder -- the sac where you store your urine in between the times you go to the bathroom.

Technologist -- the friendly person who helps the doctor and answers any questions you have.

Contrast material -- the liquid that is put into your bladder to make it look very round and dark on the TV screen so that it can be seen more clearly.

Catheter -- if you haven't guessed, this is the thin, slippery plastic tube that they use to get the contrast material from the bottle into your bladder.

Urethra -- the tube that your urine flows through from your bladder to the outside.

EXCRETORY UROGRAM (IVP)

Children's Hospital

**DEPARTMENT
OF
RADIOLOGY**

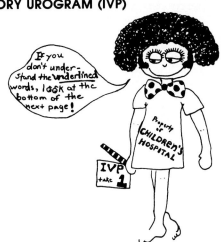

We heard you're going to have some special x-rays called an IVP done pretty soon and we thought we would tell you about them so you'll know what's going on.

The IVP is done in the <u>Radiology Department</u> of Children's Hospital. In this test the technologist will take some pictures of your kidneys. To make sure that they will come out clearly, you should not eat breakfast before the test. It will be OK to drink anything you want at home except apple juice or milk. Don't drink anything after you get to the hospital.

A <u>technologist</u> will bring you into a bright room which will be painted either blue or yellow. In this room you will see a big machine near a high metal table; this machine is just an overgrown camera. All you will have to do is lie on your back on the table and hold very still while she or he takes a quick picture. Then she or he will bring you into the yellow room right next door. Here a technologist will inject some <u>contrast material</u> into your arm. We won't kid you -- it will sting for a second as she puts the needle in. After that the rest is no sweat! It will take a couple of minutes for the technologist to inject all of the contrast material because it is very thick and she has to work pretty hard.

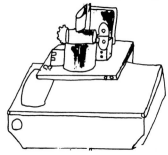

Once it is all in, she will take out the needle, put a bandaid on your arm, and take you outside.
Every few minutes you will have a picture taken just like that first one. After the technologist has taken all the films the doctor wants, you will be all done. Then all you will have to do is wait for a few minutes while your pictures are being developed. This is real service since your parents have to wait several days to have their photographs developed.

<u>Radiology Department</u> -- the place in the hospital where x-rays are taken.
<u>Technologist</u> -- the friendly person dressed in white pants or lab coat who helps the doctor and answers any questions you have.

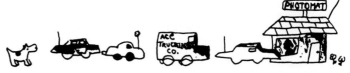

<u>Contrast material</u> -- the clear liquid that the technologist will inject into your arm that goes to your kidneys to make them stand out in the pictures since otherwise they usually cannot be seen.

ULTRASOUND

Children's Hospital

**DEPARTMENT
OF
RADIOLOGY**

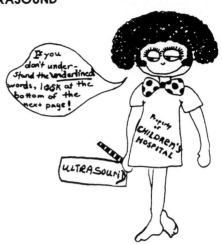

We hear that you are going to have a special test soon that uses ultrasound to see your insides. You may have heard it called an ultrasound, or an echo, or a scan, and we thought we would tell you about it so you will know what is going on. The test will be done in the <u>Radiology Department</u> of Children's Hospital.

Believe it or not, the test uses sound waves to help the doctor to look at the inside of your body. (That is why it is called ultra<u>sound</u>.) You have to believe that this is true, because no one can hear these types of sound waves. The sounds bounce off parts of your body and show where they are and what they look like. This is like the way that bats, dolphins and submarines move around without hitting things. Your doctor may want to know what your kidneys, liver, or some other part of your body looks like. For some tests you might have to drink a lot of water first and not go to the bathroom until the test is done. This is the only part that might be uncomfortable.

When it is time for you to have the ultrasound, the <u>technologist</u> will bring you into a room that has a high bed, and a big machine with a computer and a television screen on it. You will have to lie on the table, and uncover the part of your body that the doctor wants to study. Either a technologist or the <u>radiologist</u> will then do the test. There is a microphone on a long cord that he or she will use for the study.

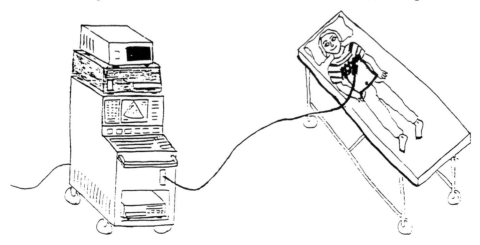

This microphone gives off the sound waves. Whomever is doing the test will squirt a lot of gooey jelly onto the microphone to make the sound move into your body better. Then all you have to do is lie still while he or she holds the microphone on different parts of your body. During the test you will be able to look at the insides of your body on the screen, but do not expect to recognize anything, because it is a pretty funny picture. You might be asked to lie on your side, or take a deep breath, or to hold your breath and not move for a couple of seconds while they take the picture of what you see on the screen. They may take quite a few pictures like this before they are done, so be patient. If you have any questions, ask the person doing the test. When they have taken all the pictures they want, developed them, and had a look at them, you are done. After you have wiped off all the gooey stuff with one of the towels they give you, you can leave.

<u>Radiology Department</u>-The place in the hospital where x-rays, CT scans, magnetic resonance and ultrasound scans are done.

<u>Technologist</u>-The person who is specially trained to do scans in ultrasound and who usually performs the test.

<u>Radiologist</u>-A doctor who is specially trained to study the insides of your body with x-rays, CT scans, magnetic resonance, or ultrasound. The radiologist telephones the doctor who asked for the test and also sends him or her a report.

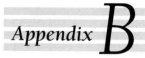

Appendix B

Patient Preparation Sheets*

INTRAVENOUS PYELOGRAM (IVP)

Preparation

No solids, milk, or apple juice the morning of the examination (or 4 hours prior to the examination).

FLUIDS OTHER THAN MILK OR APPLE JUICE SHOULD BE GIVEN FREELY.

The patient should expect to be in the radiology department for approximately 1 hour.

A sheet explaining how this examination is done should be attached. If it is not, ask your doctor for one or call the radiology department.

NOTE: For infants, skip the last feeding just before coming to the hospital. They may eat or drink in the radiology deparment *after* the examination has begun.

PLEASE ARRIVE PROMPTLY FOR YOUR SCHEDULED APPOINTMENT.

VOIDING CYSTOURETHROGRAM (VCUG)

Preparation

The patient should eat and drink normally; no special preparation is necessary. (If the patient is having both a VCUG and an IVP, please follow the instructions for the IVP).

The patient should expect to be in the radiology department for approximately 1 hour.

A sheet explaining how this x-ray examination is performed should be attached. If it is not, ask your doctor for one or call the radiology department.

PLEASE ARRIVE PROMPTLY FOR YOUR SCHEDULED APPOINTMENT.

*Courtesy of the Department of Radiology, Children's Hospital, Boston, Massachusetts

BARIUM SWALLOW (ESOPHAGEAL STUDY), UPPER GASTROINTESTINAL (ESOPHAGUS, STOMACH, DUODENUM), UPPER GI WITH SMALL-BOWEL SERIES

Preparation

Nothing to eat or drink after a light breakfast, which must be eaten before 8:00 a.m. Babies under 1 year of age may have a 9:00 a.m. feeding.

NOTE TO PARENTS AND PATIENTS: These examinations take about 1 hour, except for a small-bowel examination, which may take 4 hours or longer.

Barium studies at Children's Hospital are performed in the afternoon.

PLEASE ARRIVE PROMPTLY FOR YOUR SCHEDULED APPOINTMENT.

BARIUM ENEMA

NOTE TO OFFICES AND CLINICS: If the primary purpose of the examination is to identify a source of bleeding, an air-contrast study should be done if the child is old enough to cooperate (usually older than 4 years). SEE INSTRUCTION SHEET FOR AIR-CONTRAST BARIUM ENEMA.

Please contact a staff radiologist prior to the examination if active colitis is suspected, for acute surgical conditions, and when renal failure, diabetes insipidus, or another water-losing state is present.

Preparation

Age 0 to 2 years:	No preparation.
Age 2 to 10 years:	Low-residue meal the evening before and morning of the examination.
	See Low-Residue Diet sheet.
	One bisacodyl tablet, whole, with water, taken before going to bed.
	If the patient has no bowel movement in the morning, a Pedifleet enema should be given. This product can be purchased at drugstores without a prescription.
Age 10 years to adult:	Same preparation as for 2 to 10 years, but two bisacodyl tablets, whole, with water, are taken before going to bed.

Bisacodyl is available at the Children's Hospital pharmacy with a prescription or at drugstores without a prescription.

The entire examination will take about 1½ hours.

PLEASE ARRIVE PROMPTLY FOR YOUR SCHEDULED APPOINTMENT.

AIR-CONTRAST BARIUM ENEMA

Preparation

Low-residue diet for 2 days, then liquid diet only on the day of the examination. See Low-Residue Diet sheet.

Breakfast:	Nothing by mouth after a liquid breakfast on the day of the examination.
Age 2 to 10 years:	One bisacodyl tablet, whole, with water, taken before going to bed the night before the examination. A Pedifleet enema before coming to the hospital the morning of the examination. This product can be purchased at drugstores without a prescription.
Age 10 years to adult:	Two bisacodyl tablets, whole, with water, taken before going to bed the night before the examination. Pedifleet enema before coming to the hospital the morning of the examination. This product can be purchased at drugstores without a prescription.

Bisacodyl is available at the Children's Hospital pharmacy with a prescription or at drugstores without a prescription.

PLEASE ARRIVE PROMPTLY FOR YOUR SCHEDULED APPOINTMENT.

LOW-RESIDUE DIET FOR GASTROINTESTINAL STUDIES

Foods Allowed

Milk:	Whole, ¾ to 1 cup daily (inclusive of all milk used in cooking, or dairy products substituted for milk)
Eggs:	Soft, boiled, poached, omelet, scrambled
Meat:	Tender chicken, beef, lamp chops (well trimmed), fish. All meats should be broiled or baked.
Cheese:	Cream, cottage, mild American
Cereals:	Cream of wheat, farina, well-cooked oatmeal, cream of rice, corn meal, puffed rice, Rice Krispies, cornflakes
Cereal substitutes:	Boiled rice, macaroni, noodles, spaghetti (plain)
Bread:	White bread, soda crackers, rusk, zwieback
Vegetables:	Potatoes (mashed or well baked; no skin)
Fruits:	Fruit juices only
Dessert:	Custard, plain ice cream, junket, or pudding — limit to ½-cup serving per day; plain cake, plain cookies, and Jell-O
Soup:	Strained vegetable, broths, bouillon
Beverages:	Milk, eggnog, malted milk, frappes (within milk allowance)
Others:	Butter and cream in moderate amounts Sugar, jelly, honey, and hard candy in moderate amounts

Foods to Avoid

Fruits and vegetables, except potatoes
All fried foods
Highly seasoned foods, spices, and gravies
Coarse whole-grain cereals and breads
Hot breads, pastries, and rich cakes and cookies
Jams or preserves containing skins and seeds of fruit
Nuts and dried fruits such as raisins, dates, figs, and prunes

CT SCANNING OF THE HEAD, CHEST, AND EXTREMITIES (PATIENTS NOT NEEDING SEDATION)

CT (computed tomography) scans involve the use of x-rays with a computer to show images of structures in the head or body. An intravenous injection into your arm may be required during the examination for better definition. The examination itself is painless.

Preparation

Do not eat or drink anything for 4 hours before the examination.

Procedure

1. You (the patient) will be lying on a table. You must lie very still during the scans. If the scan is of the chest, you will be instructed how to breathe deeply and hold your breath for each image. The images are available almost immediately. The technologist will be going back and forth between you and the next room to check the images. The technologist can see you at all times and will help you if you need something.

2. A radiologist experienced in the interpretation of the examination is present during much of the examination to direct and supervise the technical staff.

3. A head scan takes 15 to 40 minutes.

4. A chest or extremity scan takes 30 to 45 minutes.

5. After the scan you will be able to resume your usual activities and diet.

6. A preliminary report is available immediately for your physician. A typed report will be mailed within a few days to your physician's office.

PLEASE ARRIVE PROMPTLY FOR YOUR APPOINTMENT. IF YOU ARE LATE, IT WILL BE NECESSARY TO SCAN ANOTHER PATIENT IN YOUR TIME SLOT, AND YOU WILL BE DELAYED.

CT SCANNNING OF THE HEAD, CHEST, AND EXTREMITIES (PATIENTS NEEDING SEDATION)

CT (computed tomography) scans involve the use of x-rays with a computer to show images of structures in the head or body. An intravenous injection into your arm may be required for better definition. The examination itself is painless.

Preparation

Do not eat or drink anything for 4 hours before the examination.

Medication

Motion during the examination blurs images, so young children (up to the age of 5 or so) will require sedation before the examination to help them lie still. The sedation may be given as an injection or as a drink.

Procedure

1. You (the patient) will be lying on a table. You must lie very still during the scans. If the scan is of the chest, you will be instructed how to breathe deeply and hold your breath for each image. The images are available almost immediately. The technologist will be going back and forth between you and the next room to check the images. The technologist can see you at all times and will help you if you need something.

2. A radiologist experienced in the interpretation of the examination is present during much of the examination to direct and supervise the technical staff.

3. A head scan will be finished 1½ to 2 hours after you arrive.

4. A chest or extremity scan takes 1 to 2 hours.

5. After the scan you will be able to resume your usual activities and diet.

6. A preliminary report is available immediately for your physician. A typed report will be mailed within a few days to your physician's office.

PLEASE ARRIVE PROMPTLY FOR YOUR APPOINTMENT. IF YOU ARE LATE, IT WILL BE NECESSARY TO SCAN ANOTHER PATIENT IN YOUR TIME SLOT, AND YOU WILL BE DELAYED.

CT SCANNING OF THE ABDOMEN (PATIENTS NOT NEEDING SEDATION)

CT (computed tomography) scans involve the use of x-rays with a computer to show images of structures in the head or body. You will need to drink oral contrast. An intravenous injection into your arm may be required during the beginning of the examination for better definition. The examination itself is painless.

Preparation

Please see Oral Contrast Guidelines.

Procedure

1. You (the patient) will be lying on a table. You must lie very still during the scans. If the scan is of the chest, you will be instructed how to breathe deeply and hold your breath for each image. The images are available almost immediately. The technologist will be going back and forth between you and the next room to check the images. The technologist can see you at all times and will help you if you need something.

2. A radiologist experienced in the interpretation of the examination is present during much of the examination to direct and supervise the technical staff.

3. An abdomen scan takes approximately 45 minutes.

4. After the scan you will be able to resume your usual activities and diet.

5. A preliminary report is available immediately for your physician. A typed report will be mailed within a few days to your physician's office.

PLEASE ARRIVE PROMPTLY FOR YOUR APPOINTMENT. IF YOU ARE LATE, IT WILL BE NECESSARY TO SCAN ANOTHER PATIENT IN YOUR TIME SLOT, AND YOU WILL BE DELAYED.

WINTHROP-UNIVERSITY HOSPITAL
SCHOOL OF RADIOGRAPHY
MINEOLA, N.Y.

CT SCANNING OF THE ABDOMEN
(PATIENTS NEEDING SEDATION)

CT (computed tomography) scans involve the use of x-rays with a computer to show images of structures in the head or body. You will need to drink oral contrast. An intravenous injection into your arm may be required at the beginning of the examination for better definition. The examination itself is painless.

Preparation

Please see Oral Contrast Guidelines.

Medication

Motion during the examination blurs images, so young children (up to the age of 5 or so) will require sedation before the examination to help them lie still. The sedation may be given as an injection or as a liquid drink.

Procedure

1. You (the patient) will be lying on a table. You must lie very still during the scans. If the scan is of the chest, you will be instructed how to breathe deeply and hold your breath for each image. The images are available almost immediately. The technologist will be going back and forth between you and the next room to check the images. The technologist can see you at all times and will help you if you need something.

2. A radiologist experienced in the interpretation of the examination is present during much of the examination to direct and supervise the technical staff.

3. Your scan will be finished approximately 2 hours after you arrive.

4. After the scan you will be able to resume your usual activities and diet.

5. A preliminary report is available immediately for your physician. A typed report will be mailed within a few days to your physician's office.

PLEASE ARRIVE PROMPTLY FOR YOUR APPOINTMENT. IF YOU ARE LATE, IT WILL BE NECESSARY TO SCAN ANOTHER PATIENT IN YOUR TIME SLOT, AND YOU WILL BE DELAYED.

ORAL CONTRAST GUIDELINES FOR CT SCANNING OF BODY, ROUTINE ABDOMEN/PELVIS

Preparation

Birth to 1 Month
Nothing by mouth for 4 hours (except oral contrast)
1 Month to 1½ Years
Nothing by mouth for 4 hours (except oral contrast)
1½ Years to Adult
Nothing by mouth (except oral contrast) after midnight for a morning examination
Nothing by mouth (except oral contrast) after a light breakfast at 8 a.m. for an afternoon examination

Oral Contrast Dose and Schedule for Administration

Preparation of Contrast Solution
Mix 10 cc of Gastrografin into 8 ounces (240 cc) of any liquid *except* milk or apple juice. (This dilutes 37% Gastrografin to 1.5%.)

Oral Contrast Regimen

Age	Dose of 1.5% Oral Contrast and Dose Intervals

Birth to 1 Month

On ward or at home:	2 oz (60 cc) the night before examination
On ward or at home:	2 oz (60 cc) 2 hours before examination
On ward or at home:	2 oz (60 cc) 1 hour before examination
In CT department:	1 oz (30 cc) immediately prior to sedation

1 Month to 1 Year

On ward or at home:	4 oz (120 cc) the night before examination
On ward or at home:	4 oz (120 cc) 2 hours before examination
On ward or at home:	4 oz (120 cc) 1 hour before examination
In CT department:	4 oz (120 cc) immediately prior to sedation

1 to 5 Years

On ward or at home:	8 oz (240 cc) the night before examination
On ward or at home:	8 oz (240 cc) 2 hours before examination
On ward or at home:	8 oz (240 cc) 1 hour before examination
In CT department:	8 oz (240 cc) immediately before sedation, or if no sedation, immediately prior to examination

6 to 12 Years

On ward or at home:	16 oz (480 cc) the night before examination
On ward or at home:	8 oz (240 cc) 2 hours before examination
On ward or at home:	8 oz (240 cc) 1 hour before examination
In CT department:	8 oz (240 cc) at time of examination

Over 12 Years

On ward or at home:	16 oz (480 cc) the night before examination
On ward or at home:	8 oz (240 cc) 2 hours before examination
On ward or at home:	8 oz (240 cc) 1 hour before examination
In CT department:	8 oz (240 cc) at time of examination

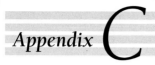 *Appendix* C

Procedure Manual

CHEST

Full inspiration and use shielding

Newborns and Infants

Use supine position until baby sits with minimal support (about 1 year old)

AP* recumbent, SID 40 inches
LAT cross-table, SID 40 inches

All Other Age Groups

PA upright, SID 72 inches
LEFT LAT upright, SID 72 inches (unless otherwise specified)

Obese Patients

Use grid

Special Views of the Chest on Request

LAT DECUBITUS—include whole chest
Right lateral decubitus is right side down
Left lateral decubitus is left side down
NONOPAQUE FOREIGN BODY—(at radiologist's request) inspiration and expiration
    or both decubiti on younger patients to demonstrate air-trapping

Portable Chest Film/Babygram

(Document the time the radiograph was taken and the technique used on portable
stickers.)

Courtesy of the Department of Radiology, Children's Hospital, Boston, Massachusetts
*AP = anteroposterior, LAT = lateral, PA = posteroanterior, CT = computed tomography, RAO =
right anterior oblique, LAO = left anterior oblique, LPO = left posterior oblique, RPO = right posterior
oblique.

AP recumbent on newborn
> Chest and abdomen should be done separately unless for line placement (umbilical arterial line and endotracheal tube). In this case, the chest and upper abdomen can be included on one film.

AP upright (if possible) on older children

ABDOMEN

AP supine—do not collimate lateral borders of abdomen

Obstruction/Free Air/Appendicitis

AP supine
AP upright to include diaphragm
If the patient is unable to sit or stand, obtain a radiograph in a horizontal ray lateral or decubitus position; left side down, right side up

Imperforate Anus/Hirschsprung Disease

PRONE abdomen
PRONE—cross-table LAT of rectum

Artificial Sphincter

AP recumbent of pelvis to include bladder and scrotum or labia
FLUOROSCOPY of pelvis—should be at same distance for each examination (check medical record)
SPOT FILMS of the sphincter; open and closed

Foreign Body

(If available, nonmetallic foreign bodies should be radiographed beside the patient to check opacity.)
Films should include area from nasopharynx to anus

AP chest and abdomen (can be done on one film)
LAT upper airway

Portable

Preferred view for neonate for free air is cross-table LAT

NECK/AIRWAY
Croup/Epiglottitis

Patient should remain sitting or upright

LAT—on inspiration, soft tissue technique
AP—on inspiration

Adenoids

LAT—nasopharynx and neck (during inspiration through nose; mouth closed)

CLAVICLE

PA upright or AP supine
AP with 15-degree angle cephalad

SCAPULA

AP
LAT (scapula lateral, patient PA oblique)

SHOULDER

AP—neutral rotation

Major Trauma

Transthoracic LAT—automatic exposure control (AEC), preselect long exposure time

Dislocation

Y view, 30- to 40-degree posterior oblique
Axillary view to include glenoid fossa, humeral head

Acromioclavicular Joints for Separation

AP—both joints on same film, upright, weights in both hands

FINGERS† (DO NOT REMOVE SPLINTS)

PA hand
LAT individual fingers

HAND†‡ (DO NOT REMOVE SPLINTS)

PA
OBLIQUE with fingers extended (use stair wedge)
LAT extended—for gross fractures or foreign body

---

†Comparison views are obtained only on request of the radiologist. It is important to image soft tissue as well as bone.
‡Initial study requires three views; follow-up radiographs of fractures require only AP and LAT.

WRIST†‡ (DO NOT REMOVE SPLINTS)

PA
LAT
OBLIQUE

Bone Age

PA left hand and wrist—radiograph of right hand if left hand is injured or obscured by intravenous line. If child is younger than 12 months, **AP** shoulder to finger tips, and **AP** midthigh to toe tips

Scaphoid—Navicular

AP with ulnar deviation
LAT
AP
OBLIQUES (both)

Stress Views for Instability

Routine—**PA, LAT, OBLIQUE**
AP—neutral, ulnar deviation, radial deviation
PA—fist clenched tightly

ANKLE†‡ (DO NOT REMOVE SPLINTS)

AP
LAT
OBLIQUE (inverted-mortise)

FEET†‡

AP
LAT
OBLIQUE

KNEE† (DO NOT REMOVE SPLINTS)

Do not use Bucky or grid, except for larger patients

AP
LAT—in 60 degrees of flexion

---

†Comparison views are obtained only on request of the radiologist. It is important to image soft tissue as well as bone.
‡Initial study requires three views: follow-up radiographs of fractures require only AP and LAT.

Trauma

AP
CROSS-TABLE LAT (for fluid level)

Additional Views

Tunnel
Tangential view—for patella

CALCANEUS†

LAT
HARRIS—axial view

TOES† (DO NOT REMOVE SPLINTS)

AP
OBLIQUE

TARSAL COALITION

AP
LAT
OBLIQUE HARRIS view

HIPS

Both sides are routinely radiographed
Both hips are not needed for comparison on postoperative radiographs
Shielding is used for all radiographs except for the following:

1. First-time females younger than 1 year; shield only one view
2. Patients with diagnosis of metastases, osteomyelitis, pelvic trauma; females with reconstruction of the acetabulum

AP
FROG LAT

Babies Having Their First Examination

Refer patients under 6 months to staff radiologist in ultrasound department to see if ultrasound is preferred.
Otherwise, obtain the following views:

AP
FROG LAT

---

†Comparison views are obtained only on request of the radiologist. It is important to image soft tissue as well as bone.
‡Initial study requires three views: follow-up radiographs of fractures require only AP and LAT.

Slipped Capital Femoral Epiphysis

AP
FROG LAT
TRUE LAT — on request

Legg-Calvé-Perthes Disease (avascular or aseptic necrosis)

AP
FROG LAT — Support each femur with 45-degree sponges

Follow-up Radiographs of Developmental Dysplasia of the Hip (DDH)

AP
FROG LAT

LONG BONES

AP both upper extremities (shoulder to wrist)
AP both lower extremities (hips to ankles)

SCANOGRAMS

1. Tape two scanogram rulers lengthwise, equidistant from the center of table such that numbers line up.
2. Position the patient supine in the anatomic position on top of the rulers such that the scale includes hips and ankles.
3. Radiograph both sides at once, unless leg-length discrepancy is greater than 2.5 cm. If the discrepancy is greater than 2.5 cm, radiograph each side separately.
4. Shield the patient.
5. The patient should not move in between the three exposures.
6. Use lead around collimated areas to prevent film from fogging.

Technique

1. Set technique according to the technique chart, starting with hip joints.
2. Using a 14- by 17-inch cassette lengthwise, with the identification nameplate at the lower edge, center the hip joints to the upper third of the cassette. Center tube to hip joints and take exposure.
3. Change to knee technique. Slide table up until the tube is centered to the knee joints. Center knees to center of the film. Take exposure.
4. Change to ankle technique. Slide table up until the tube is centered to the ankle joints. Center ankle joints to the lower third of the cassette and take exposure.

PARATHYROID SERIES OR RENAL OSTEODYSTROPHY

AP clavicle
AP hips and pelvis
AP knees
PA hands and wrists

SKELETAL SURVEY FOR POSSIBLE TRAUMA X (ABUSED CHILD) (DO NOT SHIELD PELVIS)

AP supine chest
LAT chest
AP humeri
AP forearms
PA hands
AP pelvis
LAT lumbar spine
AP femora
AP tibiae
AP feet
AP LAT skull

Films must overlap to cover all areas. Obtain additional views as needed after the radiologist has reviewed the radiographs.

SKELETAL SURVEY/METASTATIC SERIES

LAT skull (include cervical spine)
AP long bones (include hands and feet)
LAT thoracic-lumbar spine
AP abdomen (bone technique)
AP chest (bone technique)

RHEUMATOID ARTHRITIS JOINT SURVEY

Specific views as requested.

AP hips
AP shoulder
AP and OBLIQUE hand and wrist
LAT elbow
LAT knees and ankles

LEAD LINES — LEAD INGESTION

AP both knees
AP abdomen (to show recent ingestion)

SCOLIOSIS PATIENTS

PA only, or **PA** and **LAT** of entire spine, standing (unless otherwise requested).

The radiograph should include the entire spine from the level of the external auditory meatus to anterior superior iliac spines (ASIS) at a 72-inch SID on a 36-inch cassette. Collimation should include the pelvic crests. Place the Porta-Shield at the level of the ASIS. Shield female breasts with breast shields provided for patients with scoliosis (one radiograph should have been obtained unshielded). When measuring patient to determine the appropriate technique, place the calipers at the level of the breast for a male and just under the breast for a female. Close the calipers tightly and take the *inner* line measurement. Use a compensating filter, with the thickest part of the filter overlying the cervical spine region to even the density of the spine.

Scoliosis Series

Requests are for specific radiographs.

RIGHT and **LEFT AP BEND** radiographs (usually in addition to 3-foot PA and LAT) Take thoracic and lumbar bend radiographs on both sides. Pelvis should be flat when the patient bends, and the lumbar bend radiographs must include the iliac crests.

Spinal Graft out of Plaster

AP SUPINE

OFF-LATERALS—Patient is positioned laterally, then rotated forward about 45 degrees to show fusion. Center to fusion. Take both off-laterals.

CERVICAL SPINE

AP
AP open mouth (patients over 5 years of age)
LAT
OBLIQUES AND FLEXION AND EXTENSION VIEWS on request

Instability in Down Syndrome

LAT in flexion and extension with scale. The collar is placed around the patient's neck with the scale midline.

THORACIC SPINE

AP
LAT

LUMBAR SPINE

AP
LAT
Cone down L5/S1 on larger patients if lateral is not adequate.
OBLIQUES—on request

SACRUM AND COCCYX

AP 5- to 10-degree tilt cephalad, depending on age of patient
LAT

RIBS

> Erect for ribs above the diaphragm
> Recumbent for ribs below the diaphragm

PA chest (to check for pneumothorax)
AP Bucky chest (for ribs)
OBLIQUE of affected side (Bucky)
RAO — 45 degrees for left anterior ribs
LAO — 45 degrees for right anterior ribs
LPO — 30 to 45 degrees for left axillary border
RPO — 30 to 45 degrees for right axillary border

SKULL

TOWNES
AP
LAT of affected side

Neurosurgical Views — as Requested

TOWNES
AP
PA
BOTH LATERALS
Sometimes submentovertical

SINUSES

> Upright when patient is old enough to sit alone

PA (Caldwell) 15 degrees caudad center to glabella
WATERS (project antra clear of petrous ridge)
TRUE LAT — include nasopharynx to thoracic inlet on patients under 21.

FACIAL BONES

WATERS — upright if possible
LAT of facial area
PA
If zygoma is affected, **TOWNES** of facial area

MANDIBLES

AP
LAT OBLIQUE of each side (if possible, position patient upright, in the lateral position, with affected side to the head unit). Extend chin as if doing a lateral airway view. Keeping the patient lateral and with the shoulder against the head unit, tilt head to the head unit until it rests on head unit. The central ray should be perpendicular to the film.

MASTOIDS

CT may be more appropriate; check with the radiologist

TOWNES
BOTH LATERALS—25 to 30 degrees caudad; the side nearest the film is the side visualized
STENVERS or ARCELIN if patient is older than 2 years and is able to cooperate
STENVERS (PA)—head at 45 degrees; angle tube 12 degrees cephalad
ARCELIN (AP)—head at 45 degrees; angle tube 10 degrees caudad

NASAL BONES

WATERS—upright if possible
BOTH LATERALS—include nasal bone to anterior nasal spine (can be done on a detail cassette, using a ''finger technique'')

OPTIC FORAMINA

CT may be more appropriate; check with radiologist

PA OBLIQUE (side down)
Acanthomeatal line perpendicular to film
Midsagittal plane 53 degrees to film
Orbital rim parallel to film

ORBITS

CT may be more appropriate; check with radiologist

WATERS
PA (AP if patient is difficult to position)
LAT
CT shows blow-out fractures best

PETROUS/TEMPORAL BONES

Submentovertical
AP to show petrous bone through orbits
STENVERS or ARCELIN

TEMPOROMANDIBULAR JOINTS

TOWNES — 25 degrees caudad
BOTH LATERALS — 30 degrees caudad; open- and closed-mouth views
TMJ closest to film is the one being radiographed

SHUNT RADIOGRAPHS

Be sure to include entire length of tubing; overlap films

Ventricle-Peritoneum

AP and LAT chest
AP and LAT abdomen
AP and LAT skull

Lumbar-Peritoneum

AP and LAT ABDOMEN

Ventricle-Atrium Shunt

AP and LAT skull
AP and RPO chest, recumbent

FLUOROSCOPY OF GASTROINTESTINAL TRACT

If the patient has had a radiograph of the chest or abdomen within the last few days, check with the radiologist to see if another is necessary

Barium Swallow — For Esophagus

Preliminary radiographs

PA chest
LAT chest

Upper GI Series

AP abdomen — preliminary radiograph
After fluoroscopy — usually RAO with 30 to 45 degrees obliquity
Additional radiographs as requested by radiologist

Upper GI with Small-Bowel Follow-through

AP abdomen — preliminary radiograph
After fluoroscopy — follow-through radiographs every 15 to 30 minutes, depending on
the age of the patient, until barium reaches the ileocecal valve

Barium Enema

AP abdomen—preliminary radiograph
AP preevacuation
AP postevacuation

Air-Contrast Barum Enema

AP abdomen—preliminary radiograph
AP, PA, **BOTH DECUBITI**, and **SHOOT THROUGH LAT RECTUM**—preevacuation
    (Check with radiologist for additional radiographs)
AP—postevacuation

Enema for Intussusception

Use the Shiels device for pneumatic reduction

Gonadal Shielding

△ Male   ▽ Female

EXAMINATIONS	INITIAL, MALE	FOLLOW-UP, MALE	INITIAL, FEMALE	FOLLOW-UP, FEMALE	ADDITIONAL COMMENTS
Pelvis	One view △	△	—	—	Not for trauma, metastases, osteomyelits.
Hips: Anteroposterior, Frog	△	△	▽	▽	One view only on females under 1 year.
Abdomen	△	△	—	—	Avoid bladder and rectum.
Intravenous Pyelogram	△	△	—	—	Collimate to kidneys only on 3-minute film.
Chest	Use demi-aprons or standing shield				Absorbs scatter from edge of field.
Thoracic Spine	Use demi-aprons				Absorbs scatter from edge of field.
Lumbar Spine	△	△	▽	▽	Shielding limited if sacrum is included (females).
Sacrum	△	△	—	—	
Coccyx: Anteroposterior	△	△	—	—	
Coccyx: Lateral	△	△	▽	▽	Collimate well.
Femur: Anteroposterior	△	△	▽	▽	
Femur: Lateral	—	—	▽	▽	Use shield on males if exam is from the knee up.
3-Foot Spine	◄─────────────►				Use standing shield from anterior superior iliac spine down.
Angiography	◄─────────────►				Shield as directed by the radiologist.
Barium Swallow, Upper Gastrointestinal	◄─────────────►				Place lead sheeting under buttocks.

Radiographic Equipment

The following is a listing of the equipment used to collect the data presented in the tables. Equipment specifications that would have no bearing on the entrance exposures or calculated doses are not listed.

I. Generator (Philips SCP 80)
   A. Three phase, 80 kW
   B. High-frequency wave form
II. Table (Philips horizontal H)
   A. Elevating: 4-way float top
   B. Tabletop to image receptor distance (PID) = 8 cm
   C. Tabletop equivalence: 0.75 mm aluminum (Al) @ 100 kVp
   D. Automatic exposure control pickup attenuation = 0.3 mm Al @ 100 kVp
   E. Grid
      1. Grid ratio = 8:1
      2. 103 lines/inch
      3. Focused from 34 to 44 inches
      4. Cover and interspace material: aluminum
III. X-ray tube assembly
   A. 2.7 mm equivalent total filtration
   B. Standard source to image receptor distances (SIDs)
      1. Routine table Bucky examinations = 107 cm
      2. Routine tabletop examinations = 107 cm
      3. Vertical wall Bucky or cassette holders = 183 cm
      4. Sinus examinations = 115 cm
   C. Half value layer @ 80 kVp = 2.97 mm Al
   D. Radiation output = 13.5 mR/mAs free-in-air @ 70 kVp @ 61 cm from focal spot
IV. Wall Bucky (Philips)
   A. Grid placed stationary on front in rails to allow easy removal
   B. Wall Bucky front to image receptor distance = 5 cm
   C. Wall Bucky front equivalence: 0.4 mm Al @ 100 kVp
   D. Automatic exposure control pickup equivalence: 0.3 mm Al @ 100 kVp
   E. Removable grids
      1. Grid number 1: used for upright abdominal examinations
         a. Grid ratio = 8:1
         b. 103 lines/inch
         c. Focused from 34 to 44 inches
         d. Cover and interspace material: aluminum
      2. Grid number 2: used for chest examinations
         a. Grid ratio = 8:1
         b. 103 lines/inch

      c. Focused from 48 to 72 inches

      d. Cover and interspace material: aluminum

  V. Wall cassette holder for 36-inch image receptors (scoliosis examinations, etc.)

    A. Grid plane to image receptor distance = 4 cm; cassette holder does not have a cover between the grid and patient.

    B. Grid

      1. Grid ratio = 10:1

      2. 103 lines/inch

      3. Focused from 60 to 72 inches

      4. Cover and interspace material: aluminum

  VI. Upright cassette holder mounted on tabletop (upright chest examinations of children ages 1 to 5 years)

    A. Holder has no front or grid

    B. Patient exit plane to image receptor distance = 2 cm

 VII. Image receptor and processing

    A. Nominal 400-speed image receptor (routine work)

      1. Film (Kodak TML)

      2. Screens (Kodak Lanex regular)

      3. Cassettes

        a. Kodak X-Omatic cassettes

        b. Cassette front equivalence: 1.7 mm Al @ 100 kVp*

    B. Nominal 100-speed image receptor (extremities)

      1. Film (Kodak TML)

      2. Screens (Kodak Lanex fine)

      3. Cassettes

        a. Kodak X-Omatic cassettes

        b. Cassette front equivalence: 1.7 mm Al @ 100 kVp*

    C. Nominal 1100-speed image receptor (all examinations are done with 36-inch image receptors)

      1. Film (Kodak TMH)

      2. Screens (Kodak Lanex fast)

      3. Cassettes: Spectroline

    D. Processing parameters

      1. Developer

        a. Kodak RP X-Omat developer

        b. Immersion time: 24 sec

        c. Temperature: 35° C

        d. Replenishment rate: 65 cc/film

      2. Fixer

        a. Kodak RP X-Omat fixer

        b. Temperature: 32°C

        c. Replenishment rate: 85 cc/film

*Personal communication, Ken Huff and Phillip C. Bunch, Kodak Health Sciences Division, Eastman Kodak Co., Rochester, New York, 6/93.

Index

Note: Page numbers in *italics* refer to illustrations; page numbers followed by t refer to tables.

ISBN 0-7216-4534-8